BIOCHEMISTRY OF BRAIN TUMOURS

BIOCHEMISTRY
OF BRAIN TUMOURS

MARIA WOLLEMANN

WITH A FOREWORD
BY
ABEL LAJTHA
NEW YORK STATE RESEARCH INSTITUTE
FOR NEUROCHEMISTRY AND DRUG ADDICTION
WARD'S ISLAND, NEW YORK

UNIVERSITY PARK PRESS
BALTIMORE · LONDON · TOKYO

© *Akadémiai Kiadó, Budapest 1974 · M. Wollemann*

First published 1974 by

THE MACMILLAN PRESS LTD

London and Basingstoke

Associated companies in New York, Melbourne,

Dublin, Johannesburg and Madras

Published in North America by

UNIVERSITY PARK PRESS

Chamber of Commerce Building

Baltimore, Maryland 21202

Library of Congress Cataloging in Publication Data
Wollemann, Maria.
Biochemistry of brain tumours.

Bibliography: p. 161
1. Brain-Tumours. 2. Pathology, Physiological.
I. Title. [DNLM: 1. Brain chemistry. 2. Brain neoplasms.
WL358 W864b 1973]
RC280. B7W6 1973 616.9'92'81 73-9829
ISBN 0-8391-0716-1

JOINT EDITION WITH AKADÉMIAI KIADÓ, BUDAPEST

Printed in Hungary

to the memory of Prof. A. V. Terian

FOREWORD

Those interested in the physical properties of the world in ancient times did not trust in their ability to reach the answers through experiments. Even great philosophers tried to arrive at natural laws without experimentally testing them. Few in our contemporary society still think that we can understand nature without exploring it scientifically. In order to elucidate disease properly or find an effective cure, it is necessary to understand as much as possible the disease process and normal function. This can only be achieved with the tools of experimental science.

Mankind has marshalled large resources in recent times for the treatment of the sick. Illness and its treatment represent a tremendous expense as well as a great deal of suffering for mankind. Since so many of our present methods of treatment are inadequate, perhaps even primitive, it is surprising and sad how comparatively little effort is still expended on understanding pathological mechanisms. Understanding pathology is clearly directed towards decreasing suffering by improving treatment. But life is a unity, in health and in disease, and the understanding of pathological mechanisms can lead to a greater understanding of physiological systems. This book deals with tumours of the nervous system, and by giving us information about tumours, also enlarges our knowledge of growth and development. It is not surprising that the brain has been neglected by medical scientists even in comparatively recent times, since it is undoubtedly the most complex organ in the body, and trying to understand its function represents formidable difficulties. In spite of this, it is clearly one of the most important advances of twentieth century science that the brain, and even its most complex functions, appear to be within our understanding and experimental approach. Dr. Wollemann, in a pioneering spirit, has gathered our available knowledge of tumours in the nervous system and evaluated it. The brain is also a unity, and it is not possible to discuss pathology without discussing physiological mechanism; these are combined in an admirable fashion in the text. That efforts are pioneering means that we are not out of the forest: we begin to gather the facts, we have some leads, some ideas, we begin to see some connections. In pointing out what we know, and even more, what routes we have to explore, the present book does a great service and performs an important function for all of us in the field.

Abel Lajtha

> *"Adam:* But, ah, the end; if I could
>   that forget!
> *The Lord:* O Man, strive on, strive on,
>   have faith and trust!"
> Imre Madách: *The Tragedy of Man*

PREFACE

Eighteen years ago I entered the Institute of Neurosurgery in Budapest. I came from the Institute of Biochemistry of the Hungarian Academy of Sciences, which I left because of my interest in neurochemistry. There were no other possibilities for scientific research in neurochemistry and I was glad when Professor Terian, who came from Moscow to organise an Institute of Neurosurgery in Budapest, offered me a place in the newly founded institute. I had a small laboratory with a borrowed Warburg apparatus and use of the photometer and centrifuge in the clinical laboratory. Thus I started with poor equipment and no assistance whatsoever but was rich in self-confidence and had an abundance of human brain material. I obtained brain tumours as often as I needed directly from the operating room; and in collaboration with the pathological laboratory and the later founded tissue culture laboratory I investigated more than five hundred brain tumours, besides some other brain tissue mainly from cases of epilepsy and aneurysm.

During these years I had many opportunities to contact scientists all over the world working in similar fields. This was a great help to me and encouraged and stimulated further work. The application of the results of molecular biology in clinical medicine is, to my mind, an approach which might distract medicine from empirism. I feel that we are yet far from this objective but something has already started. Even if we cannot predict today the exact end of this process, we hope to achieve with the international power and co-operation of science the ultimate end: the welfare of mankind.

M. Wollemann

ACKNOWLEDGEMENTS

I wish to express my sincere thanks to my co-workers E. Róna, A. Nagy, F. Katona, E. Wester, L. Gazsó, F. Slowik, A. Barabás, E. Csanda, G. Szabó, G. Fényes, E. Paraicz, D. Áfra and to all neurosurgeons in the Institute of Neurosurgery of Budapest, to my co-workers J. C. Smith, C. Sutton, L. J. Rubinstein in the Montefiore Hospital, New York, as well as to L. Zoltán, Director of the Institute of Neurosurgery in Budapest, to F. F. Foldes, Head of the Anaesthesia Department and H. Zimmerman, Head of the Neuropathological Department at the Montefiore Hospital, New York. Without their help and interest this work could not have been performed.

CONTENTS

1. INTRODUCTION

Molecular biology opened a new period not only in general biochemistry but also in related disciplines. The rôle of DNA and RNA in cell division and protein synthesis, the exploration of primary, secondary and tertiary protein structure, and the discovery of the regulatory mechanisms in cell division and metabolism, deeply changed our way of thinking in life sciences. Pathological changes traceable so far only by histological methods became obvious much earlier with submolecular methods. The primary lesions of hereditary illnesses frequently revealed a lack of DNA or RNA dependent enzyme synthesis.

Tumour biochemistry started in 1930 with Warburg's publication 'The Metabolism of Tumours'. The fundamental finding of this book is that embryonic and tumour tissue have in common a high glycolytic metabolism even under aerobic conditions, in contrast to most normal tissue where oxidative metabolism predominates. The oxidative metabolism in cells is generally sixteen times more economical in respect of energy than the glycolytic pathway. The Embden-Meyerhof glycolytic pathway is phylogenetically the more primitive form. In rapidly growing undifferentiated or dedifferentiated tissue this pathway prevails over oxidative metabolism. Thirty years later modern molecular investigations revealed that the multiple molecular forms of some enzymes of rapidly growing embryonic and tumour tissue differ from the 'adult' form of these enzymes thus proving the observations of Warburg at the molecular level.

The definitive solution of the tumour problem, however, will probably not originate from the metabolic site, because these alterations are only consequences of the changed nucleic acid and protein synthesis of tumours. Probably, knowledge of the molecular mechanism of cell growth and division will provide the key to the tumour problem; the results of investigations of tumour promoting virus infections offer another possibility of solving the problem. The unique nature of primary malignant brain tumours, such as their extracranial non-metastasising character and the high incidence of tumours of glial origin (40%), urged brain tumour research workers first to investigate the characteristic features of normal brain tissue. Thudichum, 'the father of neurochemistry', had already written in 1884 in his 'Treatise on the chemical constitution of the brain': 'When the normal composition of the brain shall be known to the uttermost item, then pathology can begin its search for abnormal compounds or derangements of quantities.' In spite of the gaps which still exist in the basic knowledge of the normal composition of the brain, the high mortality rate of the brain

tumour bearing patients urges more and more scientists to concern themselves with this plague of mankind.

Research work on brain tumour metabolism started in the 1930s after
Warburg's classic findings on tumour tissues and the respiration and glycolysis of brain tumours. Histochemical methods for the demonstration of
glycogen were among the earliest works, being discovered by Raspail in
1825. Brain tumour biochemistry started with the investigation of changes
in this polysaccharide in 1918. The analysis of other brain tumour components followed rapidly, but is still not complete. Glycolytic and oxidative
activities in brain tumours were explored, and the investigation of individual enzyme activities soon followed, with the application of different
methods in slices, homogenates and tissue cultures.

The aim of a large part of these experiments was to establish differences
between malignant and benign brain tumours. Partial results could be
achieved without exploring differences in the fundamental molecular mechanism of malignant and benign cell growth, but the basic differences are still
obscure. Resolute pragmatic research is only conducted in a few places
owing to the theoretical and practical difficulties. Tissue culture is of great
potentiality since it affords a uniform cell population. Experimentally induced
brain tumours in animals are also useful. The chance of solving the tumour
problem in the near future is provided by the great theoretical advances in
molecular biochemistry and the application of modern methods. It is our
duty to make the best of these opportunities.

1.1. HISTOLOGICAL CHARACTERISTICS OF BRAIN TUMOURS,
EXPERIMENTAL BRAIN TUMOURS
AND BRAIN TUMOUR TISSUE CULTURES

Brain tumour research workers should be well instructed in histopathology
and neurochemistry. For those who are not trained in one of these fields,
a brief summary of the histopathology of brain tumours and the neurochemistry of brain tissue is given in order to provide an understanding of
the basic principles of both disciplines. The reader who is interested in a
more detailed description will find a list of appropriate textbooks in the list
of references.

There have been several classifications of brain tumours since the famous
scheme of Bailey (1933). At present the most generally accepted classification is that of Zülch (1962).

In order to understand the metabolic deviations of brain tumours they
are classified according to the type of normal tissue from which they originate. According to this arrangement two big tumour groups exist in nervous
tissue, one of neuroectodermal and one of mesenchymal origin. The tumours
of neuroectodermal origin include neoplasms of glial and neuronal origin.
The glioma group is generally localised in the CNS and the neuronal group
in the peripheral nervous system. The latter should generally not be designated 'brain tumour'. Tumours of mesenchymal origin can also be grouped
into several classes. Meningiomas are meningeal neurinomas of fibroblastic

or neurilemmal origin. In the latter case they should be classified among the neuroectodermal tumours. Primary sarcomas represent a third group of malignant brain tumours of mesenchymal origin. The classification of medulloblastomas among the two main groups or among glial or neuronal tumours is still a matter for discussion for reasons described later.

There are several groups of the so-called 'brain tumours' which are not included in this list. Among these are craniopharyngiomas, hypophysis adenomas, metastatic carcinomas of ectodermal origin and haemangiomas of mesenchymal origin. They are not representatives of primary brain tumours but rather of maldevelopment, for instance, craniopharyngioma; some of them occur primarily in other organs as adenoma, haemangioma and carcinoma. We shall refer to them only in special cases, comparing or differentiating them from other brain tumours (see Table I).

TABLE I

Classification of tumours of the nervous system according to their origin and malignancy

1. Tumours of neuroectodermal origin

a. Glial origin: spongioblastoma ependymoma astrocytoma oligodendroglioma glioblastoma*	*b.* Neuronal origin: pheochromocytoma ganglioneuroma neuroblastoma*

medulloblastoma ?*

2. Tumours of mesenchymal origin

a. Neurilemmal origin: neurinoma	*b.* Meningeal origin: meningioma

c. Primary sarcoma*
medulloblastoma ?*

* malignant.

Another important factor in the study of the metabolism of brain tumours is the problem of malignancy. The boundary between the malignant and benign gliomas is not as well defined as it is implied in Table I. Extracranial metastatic phenomena do not occur in primary brain tumours. The criteria of malignancy are mainly tumour growth velocity and the typical histological features of malignant growth; the appearance of mitosis and polymorphism in the cell nuclei, highly anaplastic tumour glial cells and multinucleated giant cells, infiltration and endothelial hyperplasia of the small blood vessels and necrotic areas in the centre of tumours are some of the more frequently observed malignant changes. Transformations from benign into malignant forms especially in the glioma group are not uncommon. Metabolic investigations of gliomas are important because biochemical changes due to malignancy are often manifested earlier than histological alterations. A constant feature in the course of the histological examinations of gliomas is the appearance of reactive astrocytomas and phagocytic cells such as macrophages and cells of microglial origin (Friede 1964, Rubinstein and Smith 1962). These cells should be regarded as a nonspecific defence reaction of the brain tissue against all kinds of chronic endogenous and exogenous injuries. For example, the implantation of neutral foreign bodies causes similar changes. The phagocytic character of these cells is revealed not only by their relatively high oxidative and glycolytic metabolism, but also by their elevated lysosomal degradative activity (Wollemann *et al.* 1965, Wollemann 1970). These findings support the importance of cytochemical investigations in brain tumour research, complemented by differential centrifugation and histochemical and electronmicroscopical methods.

Representatives of the glioma group may be induced by the implantation of methylcholanthrene or injection of methylnitrosourea in mice or rats. The type of gliomas developed in the brain depends on the site of implantation. The need for a reproducible source of material for biochemical research and chemotherapeutical experiments stimulated these efforts. The same object was achieved by tissue culture of brain tumours, which had the advantage of a fairly homogeneous cell population and the disadvantage of a limited quantity of cells. Similar factors are even more valid for the cytochemistry of individual cells, with the added disadvantage of losing part of the neuropil during the microdissection.

The special methods applied to brain tumour biochemistry are principally the same as those used in the investigation of normal brain tissue. Therefore, the development of these methods will be briefly reviewed in the following section on the metabolic characteristics of normal brain.

1.2. SOME CHARACTERISTICS OF NORMAL
BRAIN METABOLISM

During the last fifty years an increasing amount of data became available on the differences between the components and metabolism of brain and other organs. Differences based on functional adaptation will be considered first because these are expected to change most in tumours.

1. Carbohydrates

One of the most characteristic features of brain tissue is the high rate of consumption of glucose and oxygen due to the high rate of aerobic glycolysis. The respiratory quotient of the cerebral grey matter is 1.0, which indicates an exclusive carbohydrate oxidation in contrast to the value of 0.86 for white matter. Neurones oxidise mainly glucose and glutamic acid, whereas glial cells are capable of fatty acid oxidation and glycogenolysis as well. Glycogen was identified histochemically in the oligodendroglia and around the synapses of certain neurones. Acid mucopolysaccharides are important constituents of astrocytes and nerve cell perikarya as they play a rôle in water and ion-binding.

2. *Lipids*

Lipids constitute 50% of the dry weight of brain, which is therefore the richest organ in this material. The white matter contains more lipids than the grey because lipids form the myelin sheaths of nerve fibres and tracts. In addition to cholesterol, the carbohydrate containing lipids (glucosphingosides) such as gangliosides, cerebrosides and strandin, and the phosphorus containing phospholipids such as cephalin, plasmalogen, diphosphoinositide and sphingomyelin are all important constituents of the nerve and glial cell membranes of subcellular particles. According to earlier investigations (Fewster and Mead 1968) the ganglioside content of nerve cells is five to six times greater than that for the glial cells. However recently, Norton and Podulso (1971) presented evidence that gangliosides are glial constituents.

Lysosomes and synaptic vesicles are ganglioside containing subcellular particles. The rapid turnover of phospholipids and their regulation by different neurotransmitters is an indication of their active rôle in neurotransmission, cell permeability and specific binding of different neurohormones.

3. *Proteins*

The protein content of brain is similar to that of other organs. In the last few years, owing to new protein separation methods such as immune and gel electrophoresis, several brain protein fractions have become known which are characteristic of nervous or glial cells. These are acidic proteins of the prealbumin fraction B 10 and S-100 occurring in glial cells and nerve cell nuclei and 1342 localised in neurones. Functionally they are probably involved in specific brain functions such as learning.

4. *Nucleic acids*

Relatively less is known of the cerebral nucleic acids. The important results achieved in the molecular biology of nucleic acids were obtained from work on bacteria and virus and the most investigated mammalian tissues were liver and blood cells. Only a small amount of analytical work was carried out on nervous tissue. The highly specialised heterogeneous cell population of neurones and glial cells makes evaluation of the results very difficult. Two types of neuroglial cell nuclei have been observed in the normal human cerebellar cortex, one diploid and the other tetraploid. The tetraploid type was either in oligodendroglia or astrocytes. Reactive astrocytes are also tetraploid. From autoradiographic labelling experiments with ^{3}H thymidine and from tissue cultures, it was concluded that neuroglial cells are constantly formed from spongioblasts and that astrocytes are formed from oligodendrocytes.

RNA was first observed by Nissl in 1892 as a degenerating chromidial substance after the section of an axon. The chemical identification of

RNA was established only in 1940 after treatment with ribonuclease which caused the disappearance of the Nissl bodies (see page 121). The Casperson–Hydén school applied ultraviolet microspectrophotometric methods to measure directly the nucleic acid content of nerve cells. The rôle of nucleic acids in normal brain became interesting when Hydén (1959) and McConnel et al. (1959) suggested their possible function in learning and memory. After detailed investigations of the rôle of nucleic acids in cell replication and protein synthesis in viruses, bacteriophages, bacteria, and mammalian blood and liver cells, modern methods were applied to the investigation of brain nucleic acids. Some peculiarities of brain nucleic acids were observed, for instance, the extreme lability of certain messenger RNA-ribosome complexes (Zomzely et al. 1968, Appel 1967).

On the basis of phosphorus determinations in DNA and RNA, Logan et al. (1952) concluded that grey matter contained more RNA and less DNA than white matter. From a comparison of the RNA content of an oligo-dendroglial cell and a nerve cell in the Deiter's nucleus of the same volume and dry weight, Hydén and Pigón (1960) found 120 pg RNA in the glial cell and 1545 pg in the nerve cell. Hydén and Egyházi (1963, 1964) also established base differences between neurones and glial cells which became reversed during different learning and training situations. The adenine/uracil ratio of the glial RNA increased significantly while the cytosine decreased, but the values for base determinations differ from those given by other authors (Mahler et al. 1966, Frontali 1959) and do not fit with base pairing.

According to Jacob et al. (1966), the highest content of nucleic acids in the human brain is in the subfornical organ and pineal gland. Since neurones contain relatively more RNA than glia, the RNA/DNA index is higher in the neurone-rich parts. The RNA/DNA ratio increases during development.

A sensitive method used by the Scandinavian School for the determination of proteins and lipids in individual neurones is X-ray absorption histo-spectroscopy. Autoradiography with tritium-labelled amino acids helped to elucidate the sites of RNA directed protein synthesis. The base determinations of RNA indicated different ratios between neurones and glial cells. These differences change during brain activity, such as electrically or chemically induced excitation and learning processes. Further experiments on the molecular basis of memory and learning should soon solve these very interesting problems.

5. Minerals

Ionic equilibrium is one of the most important factors in nerve excitation, since the influx of sodium and efflux of potassium produces the action potential. Other important ions in brain metabolism are Ca^{2+}, Mg^{2+}, Cu^{2+} and Fe^{2+} and the anions PO_4^{3-}, Cl^-, and SO_4^{2-}. After changes in ionic concentration, cultured astrocytes showed increased dehydrogenase activities. It was therefore suggested that astrocytes play a rôle in sodium transport in the brain.

6. Enzymes

After reviewing briefly the normal components of brain tissue, some characteristic features of normal brain metabolism will be considered. Warburg (1930) observed that the Pasteur effect was suspended in normal brain tissue, that is glycolysis proceeds under aerobic conditions. Anaerobic glycolysis is normally present in glial cells and increases during nerve activity or electrical stimulation as well as oxidation. According to Hydén (1962), succinic dehydrogenase and cytochrome c oxidase activities increase in the neurone during vestibular stimulation and decrease in the glial cells, whereas the reverse is true of the glycolytic activity. The enzymes of the hexosemonophosphate shunt prevail in the oligodendroglia whereas Krebs cycle enzymes are dominant in the neurones. Characteristic enzymic changes take place in the so-called reactive astrocytes which will be discussed later in detail. Carbonic anhydrase activity was also located mainly in the glial cells using the Cartesian microdiver technique of Giacobini (1962). The localisation of this enzyme seems to support the carbon dioxide transport function of glial

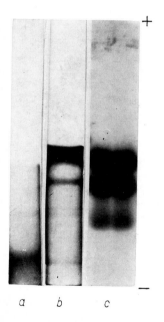

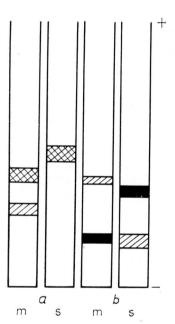

Figure 1.1. Crystalline LDH isoenzymes from swine muscle (*a*) and beef heart (*b, c*). LDH activity stained after the method of Dewey and Conklin (1960). Disc gel electrophoresis was performed according to Davis (1964) (*a, b*), starch gel electrophoresis according to Smithies (1959) (*c*)

Figure 1.2. Malate dehydrogenase isoenzymes from normal human (*a*) and rat brain (*b*). Mitochondria (m) and supernatant (s); cell fractionation was performed according to the method of Brody and Bain (1952). Mitochondrial enzymes were solubilised with Triton-X. MDH activity was stained according to Thorne *et al.* (1963)

2*

cells between the blood vessels and neurones. New biochemical methods
based on the separation of neurones and glia promise new results in the
metabolic investigation of glia and neurones (Rose 1969).

Only two enzymes of the mammalian central nervous system have been
crystallised to date, ACHE and CrPK. Nevertheless, enzyme kinetic and
electrophoretic investigations have revealed some special functional characteristics. For example, brain hexokinase utilises both glucose and fructose
as substrate in contrast to muscle hexokinase which is specific for glucose.
Unlike other glycolytic enzymes, the intracellular localisation of hexokinase
is mainly mitochondrial (about 76%), whereas liver hexokinase is much less
bound by mitochondria (30%).

The electrophoresis of brain homogenates, supernatants and particulate
cell fractions revealed multiple forms of many brain enzymes called isoenzymes, which differed generally from the liver or muscle enzymes but
were similar to heart and kidney enzymes. Lactic acid dehydrogenase is
one example. This can probably be explained by the similar high rates of
aerobic metabolism of these tissues. The enzymes existing in multiple forms
in the brain are: LDH, aldolase, creatine phosphokinase, hexokinase, MDH,
GDH, G1-6-PDH, ICDH, cholinesterases, esterases, phosphatases, MAO

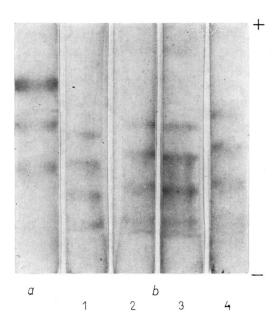

Figure 1.3. Aldolase isoenzymes from normal human cortex (*a*) and different parts of
embryonic brain (*b*) (28 weeks old); cortical
grey matter (1), white matter (2), mesencephalon (3), hypothalamus (4). Aldolase activity stained after Penhoet *et al.* (1966)

and others. Some of them, for instance LDH, are built from two types of proteins (M and H) each consisting of four subunits. This makes up three hybrid forms apart from the two original configurations, which differ in acidic or basic amino acid content (see Figure 1.1). Differences exist in the subcellular localisation of the isoenzymes too, for instance MDH has a different pattern in mitochondria and cytoplasm as shown in Figure 1.2. Another characteristic of the isoenzyme pattern is its change during development (Figure 1.3). This is common in immature tissues such as embryonic and tumour tissue.

While looking for more special functions in brain metabolism, neurotransmitter metabolism should also be mentioned. One of the earliest and best investigated enzyme systems is the synthesis and degradation of acetylcholine. Histochemical and electron-microscopical methods are available for investigating the localisation of acetylcholinesterase which degrades acetylcholine. Acetylcholinesterase is localised exclusively in the perikarya, axons and dendrites of the neurone, whereas nonspecific cholinesterases and esterases are located mainly in astrocytes. The function of the last two enzymes is not as evident as the rôle of acetylcholinesterase. Increased lysosomal activity can be traced in the hyperactivity of these enzymes and also related hydrolases such as acid phosphatase, ribonuclease, β-glucuronidase, β-galactosidase and acid proteinase. Among the other supposed neurotransmitters, indolamine and catecholamine have a separate synthesis and a common catabolic pathway. Sensitive fluorimetric methods have been published for the selective demonstration of both compounds (Falck 1962). Adenyl cyclase, the supposed β-receptor, was earlier only poorly investigated in brain tissue. Its presence in synaptic vesicles was demonstrated by De Robertis et al. (1967).

Nervous tissue exhibits a special pathway of glutamic acid metabolism, the so-called GABA shunt. The glutamic acid concentration is very high in brain (0.01 M/kg) and may serve as a unique main oxidisable substrate besides glucose. Another important function of glutamic acid in brain is the detoxicating ammonia binding capacity. Glutamic acid is thereby reversibly transformed into glutamine. α-ketoglutaric acid is also capable of ammonia binding, being transformed to glutamic acid by glutamic acid dehydrogenase (GDH) which is a key enzyme in brain amino acid metabolism. Its catalytic activity is directed towards glutamate dehydrogenation in the polymerised state and alanine dehydrogenation in the depolymerised state. Glutamic acid formation is promoted by ADP and NAD, and alanine formation by NADH and ATP. DES and GTP both inhibit GDH. Glutamate acts as an excitatory transmitter, in contrast to the decarboxylated product of glutamate. GABA has an inhibitory action on some neurones. It is transaminated in the presence of α-ketoglutaric acid to glutamic acid and SSA. SSA is oxidised in the presence of NAD and SSA dehydrogenase to succinic acid, thus arriving at Krebs cycle. By means of the GABA shunt, nervous tissue is capable of regulating the concentration of Krebs cycle intermediates.

This brief account is far from complete. It shows only some of the important characteristics of nervous tissue as related to the metabolic differences of normal glial cells and neurones. These differences are summarised in Table II.

TABLE II

Relative differences between neurones and glia cells

	Neurone (grey matter)	Glia cell (white matter)
RQ	1.0	0.86
Glucose	high	low
Glutamic acid	high	low
Fatty acids	low	high
Lipids	low	high
Glycogen	low	high
Acid MPS	low	high
Proteins:		
B 10	low	high
S-100	low	high
1342	high	low
RNA	high	low
DNA	low	high
Anaerobic glycolysis	low	high
Aerobic glycolysis	high	low
Krebs cycle	high	low
HMP shunt	low	high
Carbonic anhydrase	low	high
ACHE	high	low
BCHE	low	high
MAO	high	low
Adenylcyclase	high	moderate

2. PATHOCHEMICAL CHANGES IN BRAIN TUMOURS

2.1. POLYSACCHARIDES

1. Glycogen

The ingenious method of Raspail for staining polysaccharides in the cell with iodine was the first 'histochemical method' used by Casamajor in 1918 to demonstrate the presence of glycogen in brain tumours. The results, however, were somewhat contradictory. The early investigators (Casamajor 1918, Marinesco 1928, Kasabjan 1951) showed consistently elevated glycogen levels mainly around the necrotic areas. This elevated glycogen content was regarded originally as a sign of malignancy in the glioma group, but later astrocytomas were found to have more glycogen than glioblastomas, spongioblastomas or medulloblastomas. The glycogen content was high in the surrounding tissue of necrotic areas regardless of the tumour species. This would indicate that either the capacity for glycogen synthesis is maintained or elevated in the phagocytic or tumour cells around the necrotic parts, or that the breakdown of glycogen is diminished. In fact this is not the case; the glycogen increase in the cell should be thought of as an increase in energy fuel to compensate the lack of respiratory activity resulting from the greater vulnerability of mitochondria. In accordance with this, oligodendrogliomas are poor in glycogen and rich in respiratory enzymes localised in the megamitochondria. Fibroplastic meningioma contains relatively more glycogen than cytoplasmic meningioma or neurinoma (Friede 1957, Tajima 1960).

A much lower glycogen content and turnover were found in normal brain tissue than in brain tumours. In contrast, it was found that the glycogen content of rat hepatoma and sarcoma tissues was less than the level present in the corresponding normal tissues (Le Page 1948).

In conclusion, the relative lack of oxygen induces a decrease in the respiratory activity and a compensatory increase in glycogen synthesis in astrocytic and other tumour cells, such as fibroplastic meningiomas, resulting in the elevated glycogen content of some brain tumours.

2. Acid mucopolysaccharides

The presence of acid mucopolysaccharides in the nervous system was demonstrated by Abood et al. (1956) with histochemical methods. Acid mucopolysaccharides in brain tumours were investigated systematically first by Friede (1957) using the PAS (periodic acid Schiff reaction) histochemical method. A detailed investigation on four hundred and eighty-six intracranial and thirty intraspinal neoplasms was performed by Earle (1959). He established the presence of keratohyaline granules and mucin in several types of tumours and some intracellular granules in glioblastoma. Also areas of myxoedematous degeneration in ependymoma and central whorls in meningiomas and in the fluid of microcysts of astrocytomas were found (see Figures 2.1 and 2.2).

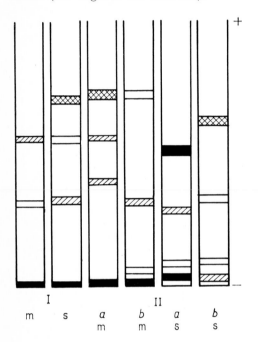

Figure 2.1. Mucopolysaccharides from normal brain cortex No. 264 (I) and from tumour surrounding tissue (*a*) and tumour (*b*) of glioblastoma multiforme No. 258 (II). Mitochondria (m), supernatant (s), MPS stained according to the method of Dagnall (1957)

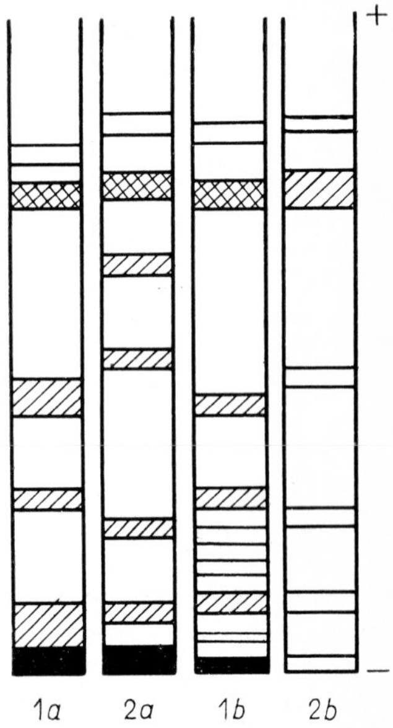

Figure 2.2. MPS from plasmocytoma No. 256 (*a*) and glioblastoma multiforme No. 258 (*b*): serum (1), CSF (2)

The normal tissue surrounding the tumour can also yield a positive PAS reaction. Similar changes were found in connective tissue around carcinomas. Friede (1957) tried to establish the chemical nature of the PAS positive substances in neurinomas. He demonstrated that it was not digested by diastase and therefore was not glycogen or starch. Tajima (1960) concluded from its resistance to digestion by hyaluronidase that it might be a glycolipid.

Recent investigations by Dorfman *et al.* (1970) using a tissue culture of glial tumour cells revealed that these cells synthesise acid mucopolysaccharides, hyaluronic acids, chondroitin-4-sulphate and heparin sulphate. Acid mucopolysaccharides were isolated from both the growth medium and the cells. The tumours were experimentally induced in rats by N-nitrosomethylurea according to the method of Druckrey *et al.* (1965).

3. Protein bound polysaccharides

Protein bound polysaccharides play an important rôle in immunochemistry. A changed pattern of mucoproteins is present in the serum in various chronic diseases. Carcinoma of the breast and lung and glioblastoma have a similar pattern in this respect. Glycoproteins containing neuraminic acid were also established in the CSF of patients with cerebral tumours (Zlotnik et al. 1959, Manno et al. 1965). The presence of acid mucopolysaccharides was demonstrated in the S-100 brain specific protein isolated from induced glial tumour cells. The increase of S-100 and B 10 glycoprotein content in glial brain tumours will be discussed later in the protein section.

These changes, as already mentioned, are not specific for brain tumours. The cerebral or serous origin of increased glycoprotein concentrations in the CSF is still not clear but their synthesis in tumour glial cell culture indicates that their origin is at least partly cerebral.

4. Glycolipids

Glycolipids reported to play an important rôle in immunological reactions have also been investigated in brain tumours. The concentration of water soluble glycolipids containing N-acetylneuraminic acid was higher in the more malignant experimentally induced astrocytomas. No difference in water insoluble glycolipid containing cerebrosides was observed in tumours and normal astrocytes (Hess et al. 1969). Christensen Lou and Clausen (1968) established the presence of dihexose ceramide in glioblastoma. This new lipid hapten, also called cytolipin H was originally isolated from epidermoid carcinoma.

The presence of a changed ganglioside pattern and concentration has been also investigated in brain tumours. Brante (1949) and Seifert (1966) demonstrated the presence of gangliosides in brain tumours which were only found in traces in normal brain. Promyslov (1966) stated that gliomas contained higher amounts of bound N-acetylneuraminic acid than mucolipids from normal grey and white matter. In contrast to these reports, Wolfe and Lowden (1964), Slagel et al. (1967) and Yanagihara and Cumings (1968) detected only a reduced amount of gangliosides mainly localised in the tumour adjacent tissue. Recently Kostič and Buchheit (1970) analysing gliomas and meningiomas by thin layer chromatography, found a lower content and different pattern of gangliosides in gliomas. Meningiomas also differed from the above tumours by having a higher percentage of galactose containing gangliosides. A mouse neuroblastoma cell line synthesised at least four gangliosides characteristic of nervous tissue. In contrast, glial tumour cell lines of both rat and human origin contained mainly haematoside as the major glycosphingolipid which is absent from the neuroblastoma (Dawson et al. 1971).

As mentioned above, glycolipids and glycoprotein act as specific tumour antigens. The antigenic property is used with success in the immunological diagnosis of tumours. By a combination of isotopic and immunoelectrophoretic methods, Cutler *el al.* (1964) and Svennilson *et al.* (1961) produced purified globulin antibodies against recidivous homologue gliomas. The immunoproteins were labelled with ^{125}I and by injection, it was possible to accurately locate the tumour *in vivo* by scintillation and make radio-autographic histological slides after excision of the tumour.

Changes in Polysaccharide Content of Cerebral Tissue in Brain Tumour

Type of polysaccharide	Type of brain tumour										
	GL	GB	AC	OG	EM	SB	MB	NN	MG	MC	TS
Glycogen	+[4]	+[2,4]	+[4]	−[4]	+[3] −[4]	+[4]	+[3] −[4]	+[1] −[4]	+[2] −[3]		
Acid muco-polysaccharides	+[5]	+[6]	+[6]		+[6]			+[5]	+[6]	+[5] +[7]	+[5]
Mucoproteins		+[7]									
Glycolipids	+[18]		−[6]								

+ = increase, − = decrease.
[1] Marinesco (1928), [2] Lipcina (1952), [3] Friede (1956), [4] Tajima (1960), [5] Friede (1957), [6] Earle (1959), [7] Zlotnik *et al.* (1959), [8] Christensen Lou and Clausen (1968).

2.2. LIPIDS

1. Phospholipids

The high lipid content of brain, especially in white matter, was known since the beginning of the last century (Vauquelin 1811). Shortly after, discoveries of the phosphorus content of some lipids in white matter were made by Couerbe (1834). He called his fraction *cérebrot* which corresponds to the present day phosphatides. He immediately suggested pathological consequences based on the different phosphorus content in the phosphatide fractions of mental cases. Although the pathological results did not prove to be long-lasting, more and more data appeared on various diseases of lipid metabolism in the brain. One of these, the Niemann-Pick disease turned out to be a hereditary illness of phosphatide metabolism.

The phospholipid content of brain tumours was first investigated by Cumings (1943). From thirty-eight intracranial neoplasms only seven contained measurable amounts of phospholipids but cystic fluids contained considerable quantities. Our own experiences confirm these observations using acrylamide disc gel electrophoresis and Sudan blue staining methods (see Figures 2.3, 2.4). Cumings attributed these changes to the degenerated tumour tissue. According to our experiments, the contribution of lipo-proteins of sera to the cystic fluid might also be partly responsible for the changes. Brante (1949) also revealed a lower lipid content in six meningiomas, eleven gliomas and three neurinomas. He concluded from the analyses that relatively low phospholipid and high esterified cholesterol values were characteristic features of brain tumours. High values of cholesterol,

cholesterol esters and free fatty acids, and a ¦low concentration of triglycerides were also reported in human mammary carcinoma (Hilf 1970).

Comparing the low phospholipid content of brain tumours with normal brain, Cohen (1955) reported that tumours contained one-third to one-half of the normal phospholipid concentration. Cumings *et al.* (1958) found small amounts of phospholipids and no cerebrosides in meningiomas, neurilemmomas and metastatic tumours from the breast and cervix. Nayyar (1963) measuring individual phospholipid fractions found a maxi-

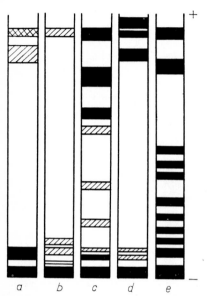

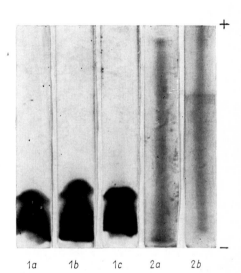

Figure 2.3. Lipoprotein fractions from lipaemic human serum No. 171 (*a*), and from serum (*b*) and cystic fluid (*c*) of neuronoma No. 138; cystic fluids of astrocytoma No. 110 (*d*), and astrocytoma No. 132 (*e*). Lipoprotein fractions stained after disc gel electrophoresis with Sudan Black, after Swahn (1953)

Figure 2.4. Lipoproteins from different parts of mitochondrial cell fractions of embryonic brain (1) (26 weeks old), cortical grey matter (*a*), subcortical white matter (*b*), thalamus (*c*); glioblastoma multiforme No. 258 (2) mitochondrial cellular fraction (*a*), supernatant (*b*)

mal decrease in cephalin and sphingomyelin. Christensen Lou *et al.* (1965) confirmed only the decrease of cephalin and not a decrease in the sphingomyelin fraction. The amount of choline was also found to be relatively high in malignant brain tumours. The relative increase of phosphatidyl-choline and sphingomyelin was localised in the microsomal tumour cell fraction at the expense of phosphatidyl-ethanolamine. Polyphosphoinositides were concentrated in brain tissue adjacent to several tumours (Kerr *et al.* 1964).

In spite of the interesting data on the high turnover of ^{32}P-phosphonositol (Ansell and Dohmen 1957, Larrabee *et al.* 1963) and its suggested rôle in nerve excitation (Hawthorne 1966), investigations on the function of this lipid in tumour metabolism are still scanty. Data on the proteolipids, which are relatively metabolically inactive, are also lacking.

The affinity of lipids to the proteins in tumours is generally decreased. According to Ambrose (1962) the high electronegative charge at the surface of the tumour cell can be attributed to a relative increase in lecithin. This impairs the contact between the tumour cells and results in the ability of tumour cells to repel each other and enables them to penetrate healthy tissue. The lack of cellular contact inhibition is proportional to malignancy. The finding that some forms of cancer are associated with failure of intercellular communication agrees well with the above observation (Loewenstein 1970).

Investigating the turnover of ^{32}P uptake into the phospholipid fractions, Selverstone and Moulton (1957) found that the specific radioactivity ran parallel with cell density, that is, it was higher in medulloblastoma and oligodendroglioma than in the less cellular astrocytoma. The ^{32}P uptake in the phospholipid fraction was measured by determining the specific activity of ^{32}P. This was shown to be 7.8–51 times higher in tumours than in the corresponding brain samples. The uptake of ^{32}P in the lipid fraction exceeded the uptake in the acid soluble nucleotide and protein fractions. It was therefore suggested by the authors that some metabolic activity was responsible for the different patterns. These observations are applied to the localisation of deep tumours in neurosurgical practice.

2. Cholesterol

Cholesterol was the first lipid isolated and identified from brain by Gmelin in 1826. It occurs in brain in greater quantities than any other single constituent except water; 4 to 5% of the fresh weight of cerebral white matter is cholesterol. In the normal adult brain it occurs in the free form, but in the developing brain some of the cholesterol is esterified (Adams and Davison 1960). In pathological cases, such as demyelination and brain tumours, cholesterol is esterified in appreciable amounts (Johnson et al. 1949, Cumings 1953, Gopal et al. 1963).

Gopal et al. (1963) found that 20% of the cholesterol was esterified in human glioma. Azarnoff et al. (1958) reported that two-thirds of the cholesterol in glioblastoma investigated was present in the esterified form and the lipid concentration was lower than in normal tissue. Sterol esters occur not only in glial tumours but also in the adjacent brain tissue (Slagel et al. 1967). Apart from cholesterol, other sterols have also been found in brain tumours (Fumagalli et al. 1964, Paoletti et al. 1965). In glioblastoma, for example, up to 4% desmosterol (24-dihydrocholesterol) and smaller amounts of zymosterol and lathosterol were also present. Desmosterol is an intermediate in the biosynthetic pathway of cholesterol. It occurs normally in foetal brain but like esterified cholesterol it disappears in the adult brain. The accumulation of desmosterol in the developing brain is considered to be due to the low activity of desmosterol reductase which is a limiting step in the foetal brain, characterised by a high rate of cholesterol synthesis (Holstein *et al.* 1966). The capacity to synthesise cholesterol from precursors such as acetate, malonate and mevalonic acid disappears in the adult brain (Azarnoff *et al.* 1958) but reappears in brain tumours (Paoletti 1963).

The reason for these phenomena might be the cellular immaturity of tumour cells or the increased myelolysis which may stimulate cholesterol metabolism. The concept of the plasmal origin of cholesterol esters was disproved by White and Smith (1968), who found a higher level of cholesterol esters in brain tumours than in blood plasma. The periods of rapid prolif- eration of glial cells could be correlated in cases of glioblastoma and oligo- dendroglioma with the increased cholesterol metabolism (Fumagalli *et al.* 1964).

After the inhibition of cholesterol synthesis with triparanol or 20, 25- diazacholesterol, the concentration of cholesterol precursors increased rapidly in mice bearing transplantable brain tumours and in the gliomas, blood plasma and CSF of patients suffering from gliomas (Fumagalli *et al.* 1966). Diagnostic importance has been attributed to this test (Vandenheuvel *et al.* 167)9.

3. *Free and esterified fatty acids*

As a consequence of the changes in lipid metabolism accompanying brain tumours the free and esterified fatty acid composition is quantitatively and qualitatively altered. A higher free fatty acid concentration was re- ported in carcinoma and other tumours (Boxer and Chonk 1960, Hilf *et al.* 1970), where it was related to the decreased α-glycerophosphate dehydro- genase activity. A characteristic of glioma sterol-esterified fatty acids was the high content of polyunsaturated acids especially octadecadienoic acid, in comparison to normal brain. Paoletti *et al.* (1961), Gopal *et al.* (1963) and Stein *et al.* (1963) investigated the free and esterified fatty acids with gas chromatography and found that in glioblastoma, astrocytoma and car- cinoma, the percentage of linoleic acid was higher than in the normal brain. Meningiomas contained a very high concentration of arachidonic acid. In contrast, the glycerol esters had a higher percentage of saturated fatty acids than normal brain tissue.

Comparing the sterol-esterified fatty acids with the corresponding blood plasma values, White and Smith (1968) reported a reduced polyunsaturated (specially dienoic acids) and a high saturated and mono- enoic fatty acid content, which together contributed approximately three-fourths of the total. Investigating the chain length of the fatty acids, it was obvious that long chain members (C_{20}–C_{26}) composed about one-third of the fatty acids, whereas plasma fatty acids contained few members of chain lengths greater than C_{20}. Therefore it was concluded as previously, that although the fatty acid composition of brain tumours differs from normal brain tissue, it is not derived from blood plasma, from which it also differs.

4. Hydrocarbons

The hydrocarbons encountered in normal brain consist mainly of the unsaturated type, such as squalene, 50 $\mu g/g$ wet weight in human brain, (Prostenik and Munk-Weinert 1963) and a homologous series of saturated branched hydrocarbons in beef brain (Nicholas and Bombaugh 1965). Squalene has been attributed with a rôle in cholesterol synthesis (Nicholas and Thomas 1959). Actively metabolising meningiomas contained five times as much squalene as normal meninges (Cain et al. 1967).

A homologous series of saturated paraffins, the n-alkanes, was also demonstrated in the same tumours by these authors. No qualitative differences were encountered between meningiomas and meninges but the proportion of the hydrocarbons was different. The authors concluded that it seemed unlikely that the hydrocarbons could be derivatives of lipid decomposition.

Changes in Lipid Content of Cerebral Tissue in Brain Tumours

Type of lipid	Type of brain tumour								
	GL	GB	AC	OG	MB	NN	MG	EI	TS
Total lipids	−2 −1					−2	+2		
Phospholipids	−2 −3					−2	+2		
[32]P uptake in phospholipids	+6		+6	++6	+6				
Sphingomyelin	+4 +5								
Cephalin	−4 −5						+2		
Cholesterol (esterified)	+2 +9	+7 +8 +9				+2			
Desmosterol, lathosterol		+10						+13	+9
Free fatty acids	+12	+11	+11						

+ = increase; − = decrease; + + = strongly increased.
[1] Cumings (1943), [2] Brante (1949), [3] Cohen (1955), [4] Nayyar (1963), [5] Christensen Lou et al. (1965), [6] Selverstone and Moulton (1957), [7] Adams and Davison (1959), [8] Johnson et al. (1949), [9] Gopal et al. (1963), [10] Fumagalli et al. (1964), [11] Paoletti et al. (1961), [12] Stein et al. (1963), [13] Fumagalli et al. (1965).

They attributed to them the function of maintaining the blood CSF barrier in the meninges. Gray (1963) also reported the presence of hydrocarbons in the lipid extracts of carcinomas. Glioblastomas contained small amounts of hydrocarbons compared with meningiomas.

Summarising the changes of the lipid composition occurring in brain tumours, a profound quantitative and qualitative alteration in metabolism is encountered. The rôle of lipids in cell metabolism and in the brain is not as clear as the function of enzymes. Certainly, since the brain tissue, especially the white matter, is rich in lipids, myelin destruction leads to increased lipolysis, but the synthesis of certain lipids is also increased in the glioma tumour cells. This might be important in the formation of the cell membrane, which consists mainly of lipids.

The low phospholipid content of tumours might also be a result of the increase of lysosomal elements, since the high rate of ^{32}P turnover indicates that the synthesis is not decreased. Phospholipase activity is mainly localised in the lysosomes (Mellorn and Tappel 1967). However, it would also be of interest to measure cytidine triphosphate concentration in tumours, considering its rôle in the synthesis of phospholipids (Agranoff 1960). The changes of another nucleotide in tumours, cyclic 3′5′-AMP, could also throw some light on the altered carbohydrate and lipid metabolism.

The consequence of the phenomenon of lipid degeneration of tumours is the disjunction of the cells (Kellner 1939). The modern experiments on the failure of intercellular communication in tumour cells complete these observations. Thus tumour cells isolate themselves from the surrounding tissue to prevent the defence reaction of the organism. The other possibility, which makes them similar to embryonic cells, is the increased demand of synthesising cell membranes. In both cases an altered lipid membrane synthesis results.

2.3. PROTEINS

1. Water soluble proteins

Proteins account for about 40% of the dry weight of normal whole brain. They are generally divided into water soluble and water insoluble fractions. The first group was investigated more exactly for methodical reasons. The separation of the various soluble brain proteins was carried out by different electrophoretic methods, such as paper electrophoresis (Palladin and Poljakova 1956), agar gel electrophoresis (Karcher et al. 1959), starch gel electrophoresis (Barron et al. 1963) and acrylamide disc gel electrophoresis (Vos and van der Helm 1967). According to the method applied, 8–15 bands have been described. Bogoch et al. (1964) published a method of subfractionation in which a combination of buffered extraction, column chromatography on DEAE cellulose and acrylamide disc gel electrophoresis separated at least one hundred different soluble brain protein fractions. This is nevertheless a small part of the estimated number of proteins occurring in the CNS.

Lipoproteins constitute a significant part of the water soluble proteins. The lipids consist mainly of cholesterol and phospholipids similar to plasma lipoproteins but carbohydrate-containing lipoproteins have also been found.

According to Swahn *et al.* (1961), the β-lipoprotein in the CSF is derived from the blood and should be considered pathological, however the presence of α-lipoprotein in CSF is normal (Dencker *et al.* 1961).

Porter and Folch (1957) described the separation of three different copper-containing protein fractions which they called cerebrocuprein. One fraction was attributed with a rôle in hepatolenticular degeneration.

The greatest variation in the protein content of different areas of brain and subcellular fractions is seen in the fast moving acidic proteins and the slower moving alkaline fractions (Davies 1970). Differences in the acidic protein content of neurones and glia have already been briefly mentioned in the introductory part on normal brain metabolism. Experiments with the acidic S-100 protein were performed in normal white matter and glial cells (Moore 1965, McEwen and Hydén 1967) and also in experimentally induced gliomas and cell cultures of these tumours (Benda *et al.* 1968, Dorfman and Pei-Lee Ho 1970). Slagel *et al.* (1969) determined the S-100 antigen using microimmuno-diffusion and found it to be present at a concentration comparable to that of normal cortex in twelve glioblastomas, one astrocytoma and one microglioma. In one oligodendroglioma the concentration was less than in normal cortex and absent or present at a very low concentration in one meningioma, one medulloblastoma and one melanoma.

S-100 was named after the solubility of this protein fraction in saturated ammonium sulphate solution. 0.5% of soluble brain proteins consists of S-100, which has a molecular weight of 24 000 and contains 30% acidic amino acids. It appears in two bands in the prealbumin fraction during electrophoresis. The faster moving band is higher in the grey matter and the slower moving one in the white matter (Filipowitz *et al.* 1968). The presence of S-100 was also demonstrated in the cell nuclei of the Deiter's nucleus by immunofluorescent methods (Hydén *et al.* 1968). S-100 has been attributed with a function in DNA regulation. However, Dravid and Burdman (1968) isolated an acidic protein from rat brain cell nuclei which was not identical to S-100. Dorfman and Pei-Lee Ho (1970) observed that the concentration of S-100 was higher in the stationary phase in tissue cultures of glioma cells than in the exponential growth phase. He therefore suggested that its rôle was not related to cell reproduction. On the other hand, experiments investigating the function of S-100 in learning processes revealed an increased synthesis in learning situations in rats (Hydén *et al.* 1970). Bovine brain S-100 protein is composed of two different subunits. There are four types of α and two types of β subunits according to Stewart (1972). Davis *et al.* (1972) demonstrated thirty-one acidic proteins in cell nuclei from rat brain by high-resolution acrylamide gel electrophoresis. They suggested the acidic proteins play a rôle in gene regulation.

A similar rôle in the learning of pigeons was attributed to B 10, another acidic protein containing hexoses which is also increased in glial tumours (Bogoch 1967). Both learning experiments were criticised by Glassman (1969) because the changes observed were not statistically significant. Acidic proteins from glial tumours were found by others (Benda *et al.* 1968, Wollemann *et al.* 1969, Dorfman and Pei-Lee Ho 1970) (Figures 2.4, 2.5)

1432 is another specific brain protein, which has a molecular weight of 40 000, and constitutes 1% of the water-soluble brain protein. It differs from S-100 and B 10 in that it is localised in the grey matter within the neurones and its concentration decreases after neurone degeneration. An increased level of 1432 has been observed in a cell culture of neuroblastoma (Grasso *et al.* 1969).

'Brain specific' proteins were also studied with antisera against normal brain and gliomas (Warecka and Bauer 1967). Hass (1966) was able to demonstrate an α_2 brain-specific glycoprotein having a high neuraminic acid content which was also present in the CSF of patients with craniopharyngeoma, intraspinal ependymoma and meningioma. However, twenty-four patients with other tumours of the CNS had none of this protein in their CSF.

Apart from being a constituent of blood, serum albumin is present under normal conditions in brain tissue and CSF. The albumin content of normal soluble brain protein is only about 5% in contrast to about 25% in CSF and 60% in normal blood serum. Oedematous cerebral cortex and white matter surrounding tumours showed an increased albumin content (Cumings 1962). Similarly, tumour tissue itself also contained higher albumin concentrations than normal brain (Gerhardt *et al.* 1963), which was probably also due to oedema. A high albumin and prealbumin content was observed in different gliomas, medulloblastomas, and meningiomas using starch gel and polyacrylamide disc electrophoretic methods (Wollemann *et al.* 1964, 1965, Monseau and Cumings 1965, Wollemann 1970). Using differential centrifugation, the prealbumin was located in the supernatant cell fraction. In one astrocytoma four fractions of prealbumin were present. The prealbumin fractions could

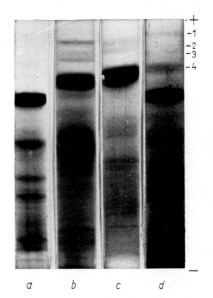

Figure 2.5. Protein fractions from supernatants of homogenates of glioblastoma multiforme No. 258 (*a*), oligodendroglioma No. 78 (*b*), spongioblastoma No. 105 (*c*) and meningioma No. 144 (*d*), stained with Amido Black B. Prealbumin fractions are numbered 1, 2, 3, 4

also be demonstrated in the cystic fluids of the tumours, which confirmed the tumoral origin of the fluid as claimed by Cumings in 1950 (see Figures 2.5, 2.6 and 2.7).

The globulin content of brain tumour tissue and cystic fluids was also changed. Gerhardt *et al.* (1963*a*) revealed an increased level of α-globulin using the agar gel method. In the cystic fluid of craniopharyngeoma, as demonstrated by starch gel and disc gel electrophoresis, heavy γ-globulin bands were present (Figure 2.8). According to Slagel *et al.* (1969) the pattern

of glioblastoma was characterised by a number of prominently stained bands
in the γ-globulin and haptoglobulin region which were not present in astrocytomas and meningiomas. These results are, however, in contradiction to
other results (Wollemann *et al.* 1965, Gerhardt *et al.* 1963a, Wollemann
1967 and 1970). The reason for these observations might be the small
amount of material examined by the authors (sixteen cases comprising:
eleven glioblastomas, two astrocytomas, one medulloblastoma, and two
meningiomas). Our material since 1963 consisted of over two hundred
tumours, and included astrocytomas and meningiomas with high γ-globulin
and glioblastomas with low γ-globulin. Conclusions based on the protein

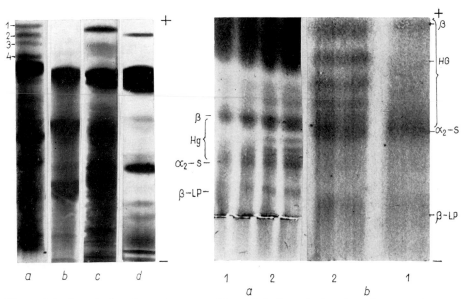

Figure 2.6. Protein fractions of
cystic astrocytomas: astrocytoma No. 84, tumour (*a*), cyst (*b*);
astrocytoma No. 272 tumour (*c*),
cyst (*d*). Prealbumin fractions
are numbered 1, 2, 3, 4

Figure 2.7. Protein fractions from cystic
fluid (1) and serum (2) of spongioblastoma
after starch gel electrophoresis (*a*); higher
magnification of β-lipoprotein, α₂-slow
globulin, haptoglobins and β-globulin fractions (*b*); note absence of haptoglobin in
the cystic fluid

pattern must be viewed with caution owing to the great variability in protein content and its distribution in tumours. No correlation was found
between the patterns of the serum protein fractions and those of the cysts
and CSF; except for cysts associated with cerebellar haemangioblastoma and
the CSF from meningitis and post-operative conditions in which blood
had been mixed with the fluids. According to Cumings (1953), an increase
in γ-globulin was present in cystic fluids, CSF and in two cases in the tissue
of malignant tumours. The sera investigated in conjunction with the CSF
and cystic fluids had different patterns (Figures 2.8, 2.9 and Table III).

TABLE III

Protein content of the different body fluids and tumours as % of total protein

Protein fractions	Sera (5) %	Cysts (3) %	Subdural haematoma (5) %	CSF (10) %	Tumours (5) %
Prealbumin	1.3– 4.3	0– 5.6	0.9– 8.1	5.6–16.2	4.2–19.8
Albumin	58.0–68.0	23.5–45.0	63.0–71.0	34.0–62.0	13.0–25.0
Postalbumin	2.2– 5.0	5.9– 6.6	4.3– 4.7	3.0– 5.7	8.3–13.7
Transferrin	5.5–10.3	12.1–16.8	5.6– 9.0	7.7–15.5	13.7–27.8
α-2s globulin	2.9– 6.7	6.2– 6.9	2.3– 4.7	3.1– 7.6	9.0–11.2
Haptoglobulin	12.4–20.7	9.5–23.5	2.4– 7.7	4.9– 7.3	12.3–20.5
β-Lipoprotein	3.5– 6.6	2.3–11.0	4.6– 7.5	5.1– 9.6	6.8–10.0
γ-Globulin	4.5– 8.0	9.2–10.3	1.8– 4.2	3.0– 8.5	8.8–18.5

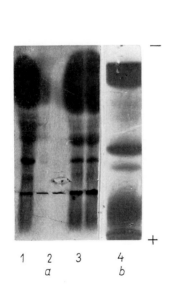

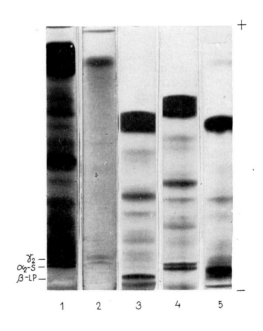

Figure 2.8. Protein fractions from serum (1), CSF (2) and cystic fluid (3, 4) from craniopharyngeoma No. 23 as revealed by starch gel (a) and disc gel (b) electrophoresis

Figure 2.9. Protein fractions from astrocytic cyst (1) and CSF (2) No. 205; note the selective increase of β-lipoprotein, α_2-slow and γ_2-globulin fractions. The same protein fractions are enhanced also in subdural haematoma fluid No. 260, left side haematoma (3), right side haematoma (4) and encephalitis No. 278, CSF (5)

The protein changes in the CSF were not characteristic in tumour-bearing patients. In 30–40% of the brain tumours there was a relative increase of α- and β_1-globulin, a decrease of β_2-globulin (β-tau) and a diffuse increase of γ-globulin (Lowenthal 1966). Using immunological methods (Ursing et al. 1962, Bauer 1966, Clausen 1966) an increase in α-macroglobulin, β-lipo-protein, M immunoglobulin and β_2-glycoprotein and an absence of β-tau was observed, which is common in meningitis, brain tumours, polyneuritis and other neurological illnesses. They should be regarded as consequences of the altered blood-brain barrier permeability. Results were published by Dencker et al. (1961) and Swahn et al. (1961) on the pathological occurrence of α_2-globulin in the CSF of brain tumours. According to Hass (1966) a glio-blastoma specific α_2-globulin appeared also in brain tumours. The fast α_2-glo-bulin band is increased in the CSF of patients with polyneuritis (Monseau and Cumings 1965). Coeruloplasmin, a copper-containing α_2-globulin frac-tion with diamino oxidase activity normally present in blood sera is lacking in hepatolenticular disease. According to Bauer et al. (1969) and Mahaley (1969) the production of γ-globulin also takes place within the central nervous system. It has been recently established that antigens from colonic cancer cells of adult humans are present in normal digestive cells of human embryos but they normally disappear after birth. The presence of embryonic constituents in malignant tumours could be explained assuming that these cells are derived from totipotent differentiated cells by derepression of the genome, for example by viruses, hormones and chemical carcinogens (Gold et al. 1968, Pasternak 1970). It would be of interest to perform similar experiments on brain tumour antigens and embryonic brain tissue.

2. Water insoluble proteins

Insoluble proteins make up about 50% of the brain proteins. The proteolipids are soluble in a chloroform-methanol-water mixture (Folch and Lees 1951) and may contain up to 50% lipids. The lipids consist of a mixture of various phospholipids. The residual protein is classically called 'neurokeratin'. Insoluble proteins can also be extracted by various treatments with deter-gents (Triton-X, digitonin, sodium dodecylsulphate), enzyme digestion with trypsin, and treatment with dilute acid or alkali.

No marked differences in the amino acid content of proteins in the brain have been revealed between benign and malignant brain tumours. According to Wender and Walingóra (1962) the cystine content was lower and the phenylalanine level higher compared with normal material.

Summarising the data obtained on the protein content and changes in brain tumours, there is little evidence of an alteration in any one of the major protein fractions. The S-100 and B 10 increase in glioma is an excep-tion, but data on the absolute increase in gliomal cells compared with normal glial cells are still unavailable. In spite of the very sensitive micro methods, such as immunoelectrophoresis and acrylamide disc electrophoresis, no consistent and characteristic changes were encountered in the CSF of tumour-bearing patients. The appearance of globulin fractions and lipoproteins is also common in other demyelinating processes in chronic diseases of the CNS.

The investigation of brain protein structure lags behind that of other tissues because only a few brain proteins and enzymes are available in a sufficiently purified form. The investigation of cystic fluid is more hopeful from the diagnostic viewpoint because it contains more information on the nature of the tumour, although it may be contaminated with blood from haemorrhages. Therefore, a comparison of the protein fractions of tumour, sera, cyst and CSF of the same patient is very useful.

A rather neglected field in brain tumour research is the measurement of the turnover of tumour proteins. Although experiments with normal adult and embryonic brain tissue, reveal heterogeneity of amino acid incorporation, particularly in neurones, glial cells and subcellular fractions, it can be concluded from indirect evidence, such as increased foetal brain and glial cell protein turnover, that the synthesis of certain proteins taking part in cell duplication may be enhanced. Possible diagnostic importance can be attributed to a changed level of protein synthesis, which, by the use of labelled amino acids in the CSF, may lead to the localisation of tumours. The uptake from the blood stream of radioiodinated human serum albumin and radioiodinated fatty acids has been studied for diagnostic purposes (Cutler 1964, Tator and Schwartz 1969). Sutton and Becker (1969) suggested peroxidase as a carrier protein for introducing cytotoxic groups into tumour cells taking advantage of pinocytosis because it is superior to the more commonly used albumin and globulin. It enters the tumour more rapidly

Changes in Protein Content of Cerebral Tissue in Brain Tumours

Type of protein	Type of brain tumour							
	GL	GB	MC	MG	EI	CP	MB	NB
Albumin	+[3]		+[2]	+[2]			+[3]	
Prealbumins:								
10-B, S-100	+[4-7]			+[4-7]	+[8]		+[4-7]	
1432	+[8,9]							+[9]
α-globulin	+[6,7]	+[1]						
β-globulin	+[11]							
γ-globulin	+[11]					+[5]		
Amino acids:								
cystine	−[10]							
phenylalanine	+[10]							

+ = increase; − = decrease.
[1] Hass (1966), [2] Paoletti *et al.* (1961), [3] Gerhardt *et al.* (1963), [4] Wollemann *et al.* (1965), [5] Wollemann *et al.* (1969), [6] Wollemann (1970), [7] Monseau and Cumings (1967), [8] Bogoch (1967), [9] Grasso *et al.* (1969), [10] Wender and Walingóra (1962), [11] Lowenthal (1966).

and a higher percentage of the protein entering the tumour is present intra-cellularly within a relatively short time after administration.

In order to understand the fundamental question of tumour formation, changes in nucleic acid content will be considered before the problem of protein synthesis and metabolism.

2.4. NUCLEIC ACIDS

The nucleic acids are perhaps the most important macromolecules in tumour genesis, nevertheless little is known about their rôle in brain tumours in comparison with what is known about polysaccharides, lipids or proteins.

1. DNA

Cumings first determined in 1943 the nucleoprotein phosphate fraction in brain tumours and cysts. He demonstrated a high DNA and RNA content in malignant tumours. Heller and Elliott (1954) systematically measured the total DNA content per nucleus in different parts of normal human brain and various tumours (gliomas, medulloblastomas, meningioma and meta-static carcinoma). They found a higher total DNA content with the highest values in a medulloblastoma. The DNA concentration in the cell nuclei of the glioma group paralleled the malignancy, but meningiomas and meta-static carcinoma also showed enhanced DNA concentrations. Cohen (1955) reported that the increase in DNA content of tumours was due to the greater cellularity of neoplasms. The ^{32}P uptake into nucleic acids was also increased and paralleled the cellular density (Selverstone and Moulton 1957). Nayyar (1963) confirmed the data on the increased DNA content of tumours. The estimations were based on the Schmidt–Tannhauser method (1945). In the brain, however, one should make allowances for the presence of relatively high amounts of phosphoinositides in the residual phosphorus fraction (Logan et al. 1952). Lapham (1959), differentiating between two types of glioblastomas on a cytological and cytochemical basis, demonstrated many large nuclei and greatly elevated levels of DNA in the 'large cell' type of glioblastoma multiforme. The 'small cell' type glioblastoma contained only small nuclei and exhibited low DNA values. When evaluating the increased DNA content in brain tumour cells, one should take into account the fact that the neurones cease to divide after birth, whereas the glial cells retain their reproduction capacity. Hence no net DNA synthesis occurs in the neu-rones after birth, in contrast to the glial cells.

2. RNA

The fluorescent cationic dye, acridine orange, has a strong affinity for nucleic acids in living and fixed tissue. When used to stain fixed tissue acridine orange differentiates between DNA and RNA, the former fluoresces green, and the latter red. In the living nerve cell DNA fluoresces green, Nissl substance orange, and other types of RNA either fluoresce green or do not stain. However the cytoplasm of certain types of neoplastic cells fluoresces orange even in the living state. Stein and Eisinger (1963) using the acridine orange staining method in gliomas showed a greater nuclear DNA activity in glioma tumour cells and a decreased RNA content in multinucleated giant cells of glioblastoma multiforme. The small capillary-like vessels of rapidly growing glioma contained RNA in their endothelial cytoplasm and they also exhibited strong DNA staining compared with static vessels. The nuclear fluorescence was significantly increased in the malignant tumours.

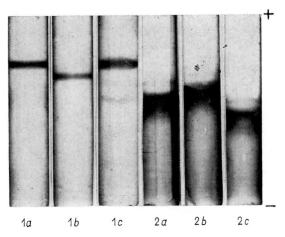

1a   1b   1c   2a   2b   2c

Figure 2.10. RNA extracted from spongio-blastoma No. 105 (1) and oligodendroglioma No. 123 (2) by the phenolic method; nuclear (*a*), mitochondrial (*b*) and supernatant (*c*) cell fractions, stained with acridine orange (1) and toluidine blue (2) according to Tsanev (1965)

In preparing cell fractions from brain tumours, high acridine orange staining of RNA was found in the ribosomal cell fractions of a spongio-blastoma and oligodendroglioma compared to the surrounding normal brain tissue as demonstrated by disc gel electrophoresis (Figure 2.10) (Wollemann *et al.* 1969).

Another trend in nucleic acid research is the analysis of base content and sequence, which is briefly called the 'code', because protein synthesis depends on the triplet base sequence of the nucleic acids. The pyrimidine–purine base pairs in DNA are thymine–adenine and cytosine–guanine. In RNA, uracil—the demethylated product of thymine—is usually present instead of thymine.

RNA is classified according to its function in the cell, as messenger, transfer and ribosomal RNA (see also page 118). Transfer RNA makes up about 15–20%, ribosomal RNA 75–80% and messenger RNA less than 5%

of the total RNA in the cell. The function of transfer RNA is to 'transfer' the single amino acids to the site of protein synthesis on the ribosomes. They contain a few other constituents, the so-called rare bases, which are generally characterised by an extra methyl group. They contain for example thymine, normally present only in DNA, 5-methylcytidine, 1-methyladenine and N-7-methylguanine. A specific RNA-methylase is associated with the avian myeloblastovirus, an oncogenic virus, which transfers a methyl group from S-adenosylmethionine to certain guanine bases in RNA to give N-2-methylguanine (Gantt et al. 1971). Viale et al. (1969), Viale and Kroh, (1971) demonstrated that transfer RNA from cerebral tumours contained more methylated bases and 2-deoxyriboses than normal human brain. In gliomas the increase of methylated nucleosides was proportional to the degree of malignancy. The primary structure of the 18 S and 28 S ribosomal RNA and also the ribosomal pattern were different in various types of tumours. The authors assume that a loss of the specificity of enzymic methylation occurs in tumours, similar to the undifferentiated embryonic tissue where the rate of base methylation is also higher.

Druckrey et al. (1965) induced experimental gliomas by intravenously injecting methylnitrosourea into rats and demonstrated that diazomethane was formed which induced brain tumours. Diazomethane acts by methylating guanine and thus changing the code. Hess et al. (1969) using the same method to produce experimental brain tumours established that in astrocytomas the DNA content exceeded all normal brain regions except the cerebellar granular layer.

A single dose of N-ethyl-N-nitrosourea in rats causes extensive degenerative changes in all types of glial cells, while neurones react less obviously to the toxic stimulus (Lantos 1971).

Chemically induced tumours grew more rapidly and contained more DNA than virus induced tumours. In polyoma virus-induced astrocytomas, differentiated cells grew more rapidly than non-differentiated cells produced by the simian virus 40 (Schein 1968). The more malignant experimental brain tumours had more RNA and higher RNA/DNA ratios. High nucleic acid and low phospholipid values were also characteristic of experimentally induced gliomas similar to human gliomas.

Kirsch (1969) explained the decrease of pentose nucleic acids in the periphery of glioblastomas as a consequence of tissue anoxia. Therefore he also gave them an energy reserve function. The increased hexosemonophosphate shunt activity of the glial tumours also effects an increased pentose supply for the synthesis of nucleic acids.

Ikuta and Zimmermann (1964) using carcinogenic hydrocarbons (methylcholanthrene, dibenzanthracene and benzpyrene) for inducing brain tumours in mice by pellet implantation, observed in the reactive cells of most animals during the pre-cancerous stage cylindrical rods or filaments with a transverse diameter of 170 Å. The particles disappeared with the development of neoplasms. They had morphological similarities to viruses but were not identical with any of them. They consisted of RNA and protein. The authors assumed that they were produced by the endoplasmic reticulum as a result of stimulation by the chemical carcinogens.

Summarising the changes in nucleic acid content, high amounts have been found especially in malignant brain tumours, as well as an increase in the ratio of methylated bases. These alterations reflect an abnormally increased cell replication and protein synthesis.

As for the aetiology of brain tumours especially that of malignant tumours, there is still a gap in our knowledge on the mechanism of cell multiplication. Carcinogenic substances as well as viruses are active tumour inducers. Among the first group, carcinogenic activity is attributed to alkylating agents which react preferentially with the guanine residue of DNA (Brookes and Lawley 1961, Druckrey *et al.* 1965). Pullmann and Pullmann (1965) assumed that the carcinogenic activity of the polycyclic hydroc‚arbons was associated with the electron distribution in the active molecules which may act by producing mutagenesis of DNA. The oncogenic viru   may act by inducing specific DNA configurations of its own RNA andla DNA template (Dulbecco 1967). Other mechanisms such as loss of regulatory proteins as proposed for the β-galactosidase lac operon in *E. coli* by Jacob and Monod (1965), as well as carcinogenic activity at the level of protein synthesis should be also taken into consideration as tumour producing possibilities.

Changes in Nucleic Acid Content of Cerebral Tissue in Brain Tumours

Type of nucleic acids	Type of brain tumour								
	BT	MT	GL	GB	AC	OG	SB	MG	MC
DNA	$+$[1]	$-$[1]	$+$[3]	$+$[5]				$+$[3]	$+$[3]
^{32}P uptake in nucleic acids			$+$[2] $+$[6]						
RNA	$-$[1]	$+$[1]			$-$[6]	$+$[8]			
tRNA			$+$[7]						
Methylated RNA			$+$[9]						
Ribosomal RNA						$+$[4]	$+$[4]		

+ = increase; − =decrease
[1]Hess *et al.* (1969), [2]Selverstonn and Moulton (1957), [3]Heller and Elliott (1954), [4]Wollemann *et al.* (1969, [5]Lapham (1959), [6]Stein *et al.* (1963), [7]Viale *el al.* (1969), [8]Kirsch (1969) [9]Druckrey *et al.* (1965).

2.5. MINERALS

The discharge of the nerve cell and the conduction of the nerve impulse along the nerve fibre are linked with the passage of electrolytes across cell membranes. The tissue cells are generally high in K^+ and PO_4^{3-} and low in Na^+ and Cl^-. The composition of the extracellular space in contrast is low in K^+ and PO_4^{3-} and high in Na^+ and Cl^-. In brain, however, the chloride concentration is relatively high compensating for the excess of cations consisting mainly of K^+. The anion deficit is compensated also by amino acids, acid mucopolysaccharides, lipids, proteins and nucleic acids. Regarding the mineral distribution, sodium, potassium, copper, iron, calcium, magnesium and manganese are relatively evenly distributed between grey and white matter in contrast to phosphorus, which occurs in higher concentrations in white matter than in grey matter.

Cumings (1943) studied the K^+, Na^+, Cl^-, Ca^{2+}, PO_4^{3-} and water content of brain tumours and cysts. The only significant differences were in the distribution of the phosphate fractions. The phospholipid content was low, but the acid soluble phosphorus and nucleoprotein phosphorus were high. Graschenkov and Hekht (1960) found a high concentration of Cu^{2+} and Ca^{2+} in cerebral tumours and Selverstone and Moulton (1957) measured an increased ^{32}P and ^{42}K uptake in gliomas. Canelas et al. (1968) investigated the Na^+, K^+, Ca^{2+}, PO_4^{3-}, Mg^{2+}, Cu^{2+} and SO_4^{2-} content of astrocytomas, glioblastomas and medulloblastomas. A higher Ca^{2+} content was present in every tumour. The Cu^{2+} content was parallel to malignancy and the Mg^{2+}, Cu^{2+} and SO_4^{2-} concentrations were high in the peritumoural tissue. The Na^+, K^+, Cl^- and SO_4^{2-} contents were higher in the benign astrocytomas than in the medulloblastomas and glioblastomas.

Changes in Ion Content of Cerebral Tissue in Brain Tumours

Type of ion	Type of brain tumour					
	MT	GL	GB	AC	MB	TS
^{32}P uptake		$+$[1]				
^{42}K uptake		$+$[1]		$+$[3]		
Cu^{2+}	$+$[3]	$+$[2]				$+$[3]
Ca^{2+}	$+$[2]	$+$[3]	$+$[3]		$+$[3]	
Mg^{2+}		$+$[3]	$+$[3]		$+$[3]	$+$[3]
SO_4^{2-}		$+$[3]	$+$[3]		$+$[3]	$+$[3]

$+$ = increase.

[1] Selverston and Moulton (1957), [2] Graschenkov and Hekht (1960), [3] Canelas et al. (1968).

3. METABOLIC CHANGES IN BRAIN TUMOURS

3.1. GENERAL INFORMATION ON ENZYMES AND TUMOUR METABOLISM

After a brief description of the components which make up brain tumours, the process by which these substances are synthesised and degraded will be examined. The enzymes have a vital function in the organisation of this metabolism, and they will therefore be considered according to their function.

The enzymes are all proteins. They contain active sites for the binding of substrate which is converted into product. By binding substrate (or substrates) at their surface and catalysing product formation they lower the activation energy of the chemical reaction, which would otherwise require a temperature not compatible with the living organism. To obtain their full activity enzymes require certain well-defined conditions, that is, optimal pH, temperature, substrate and ion concentrations and the addition of cofactors. Under certain conditions the enzymes may act reversibly, which means that they can convert their product back into substrate. By the addition of certain compounds it is possible to enhance or inhibit the activity of enzymes. Many drugs, for example chemotherapeutic agents and antibiotics, act in this way.

The enzymes are localised in different parts of the cells according to their functions. For example, oxidative enzymes are mainly localised in mitochondria, glycolytic enzymes in the cytoplasm, protein-synthesising enzymes in the ribosomes; enzymes synthesising neurotransmitters in the synaptosomes, and enzymes building nucleic acids in the cell nucleus.

The enzyme activities are generally regulated by the endproduct, which is produced in a subsequent series of enzyme reactions. This kind of regulation is called *feedback inhibition*. The product of the last reaction inhibits the first enzyme of the system, not at the substrate binding site but generally at another, that is, 'allosteric' site, by changing the configuration of the enzyme. It seems very likely that some of the regulatory mechanisms of cell division are altered in tumour cells.

Oxidative and glycolytic enzymes will be first considered in a partly historical manner, followed by enzymes of lipid, amino acid, protein and nucleic acid metabolism, and concluding with the hydrolytic enzymes. Before starting with detailed mechanisms, some general features of brain respiration and glycolysis, and the enzymes involved, will be considered.

Since Warburg introduced his manometric technique in 1923, efforts have repeatedly been made to measure tissue slice respiration and glycolysis in various animals and organs and more specifically in different parts of the same organ and different individual cells. Because the brain is a highly specialised organ with different types of cells, respiratory and glycolytic rates were measured at different sites; they were found to be characteristic, depending on the region and the cell population. White matter, for example, respires at half or less the rate of grey matter, but white matter is poor in cells. The individual average cell respiration in white matter is higher than the average cell respiration in cerebral cortex, according to Heller and Elliott (1955). Among glial cells oligodendroglia are more active than astrocytes. Neurones are responsible for at least 70% of the respiration of the cerebral cortex.

As noted previously, the brain under normal physiological conditions uses glucose almost exclusively as the substrate for respiration (see page 16). The glucose is metabolised almost entirely by the Embden–Meyerhof glycolytic pathway. In normal conditions the hexosemonophosphate shunt is of little importance. Under aerobic conditions the pyruvate formed from glucose in the glycolytic cycle is oxidised in the tricarboxylic acid cycle to carbon dioxide and water. The only amino acid which partly supports brain respiration is glutamic acid.

Brain tissue is capable of aerobic glycolysis. It produces through a series of enzymic reactions two molecules of lactic acid from one molecule of glucose. The energy yield per glucose molecule is only two mols of high energy phosphate bond, while the complete oxidation of glucose to carbon dioxide produces thirty-eight units of high energy phosphate bond. White matter has a lower glycolytic activity than grey matter.

Tissues capable of anaerobic glycolysis are usually inhibited under aerobic conditions. This suppression of glycolysis is called the Pasteur effect, since Pasteur discovered that the production of alcohol in yeast cells is depressed under aerobic conditions. Active aerobic glycolysis has been observed with brain cortex slices, but the rate decreases on incubation under aerobic conditions with a small accumulation of lactic acid. Anaerobic glycolysis is a major source of energy in the brain of embryonic and newborn animals.

In dealing with the respiration and glycolysis of tumours one cannot ignore the pioneer work of Otto Warburg in the 1920's which is summarised in his monograph 'The Metabolism of Tumours' (1930). By applying his newly-developed manometric method to the study of tumour metabolism, he established the high aerobic and anaerobic glycolysis of tumour slices. In normal tissue the anaerobic glycolysis is usually lower than that of tumours of the same organ. Normal tissue displaying high aerobic glycolysis similar to tumours are: jejunal mucosa, renal medulla, retina, leukocytes, embryonic cells and some virus-infected cells.

The overall respiratory rate of tumour slices is very variable and is in general similar to the oxidative rate of normal tissues (Aisenberg 1961).

In connection with the metabolism of brain tumours, Victor and Wolf (1937) were the first to measure the aerobic and anaerobic respiratory and glycolytic activities in biopsy specimens. They found a low oxygen uptake in glioblastoma, astrocytoma and medulloblastoma and a relatively high respiratory rate in oligodendroglioma. The glycolytic activities were higher than the oxygen uptake of tumours, which is characteristic of tumours in contrast to brain tissue. Large variations were present among the same cell types in tumours. This was also reflected in the metabolic activity of the same types of tumours.

Heller and Elliott (1955) confirmed the results of Victor and Wolf (1937) and extended the previous investigations to ten brain tumours (two medullo-blastomas, two glioblastomas, a malignant glioma, four astrocytomas and one oligodendroglioma). They established that on a wet weight basis, the oxygen uptake was about the same in gliomas, medulloblastomas and white matter, with the exception of oligodendrogliomas, where it was higher; but when stated per cell number the respiration in tumours was invariably lower than that in cerebral cortex or white matter. Anaerobic glycolysis was also low in the tumours, but as noted previously, higher than respiration, which is characteristic of tumour and embryonic tissue. According to the authors, differences in respiration between oligodendroglioma and astrocy-toma reflect the normally higher respiration of oligodendroglial cells com-pared to the lower respiration of the normal astroglia. The malignant gliomas revealed a relatively high glycolytic activity.

McIlwain (1959) investigated metabolic responses to electrical impulses in normal brain tissue and cerebral tumour slices. The metabolic increase after electrical stimulation was low or absent in tumours. This can only be explained by the low respiratory activity, because glycolysis in the tumours investigated was high. Similar changes were reported in foetal and pro-liferating glial tissue. According to Himwich (1951) the lower metabolic rate of cerebral tumours can be correlated with the reduced cerebral blood flow but other factors must also be present because reduced oxygen consumption and blood flow appear only later in the necrotic centre of tumours.

High lactate and normal glutamate levels were measured by Lehrer (1962) in all types of tumours. Steady-state levels of lactate, ADP and AMP were higher, and ATP and CrPK were lower in chemically induced ependymo-blastoma than in brain, but changes were only obvious in the malignant part of the tumours where the blood supply was sufficient (Maker *et al.* 1969). According to Shrivastava and Quastel (1962) tumour cells will invade and proliferate in those regions where nutritional conditions are optimal and where substances such as glutamine, which have a controlling effect on tumour growth, become available as a result of glucose deprivation.

A new and interesting approach to the genesis of tumours in molecular terms attributable to a decline mechanism of enzyme regulation is given by Weber and Lea (1965). Differentiating between slowly, moderately and rapidly growing hepatomas, they stated that a decrease of gluconeogenesis and an increase of glycolysis and glucose oxidation parallels the increase in growth rate. Together with the decrease of glucogenetic enzymes their induction with steroids also ceases. A similar pattern could also be outlined for the slow and rapid growth in brain tumours.

3.2. GLYCOLYTIC ENZYMES

After the general review of brain and tumour glycolysis the individual enzymes concerned in glycolysis will be briefly discussed. The general scheme of glycolysis is similar in cerebral and tumour tissue (see Figure 3.15), although differences in enzyme structure and action are encountered among the single enzymes which are examined in detail below.

1. Glycogen breakdown and synthesis

Phosphorylase is normally present at high levels in cerebral tissue, as demonstrated by Cori *et al.* (1938). It exists in two principal forms, '*a*' and '*b*'. Phosphorylase *a* is the more active phosphorylated form and *b* the non-phosphorylated, less active, enzyme. The transformation of *b* to *a* is a complicated process involving several other enzymes (phosphorylase kinase and phosphorylase kinase-kinase) and cofactors (3'5'-cyclic AMP, ATP, Mg^{2+}) which are all necessary for the transformation. Pyridoxal phosphate, AMP, glycogen and SH groups play a rôle in the molecular transitions (Helmreich 1970), (see Figure 3.1).

The action of phosphorylase is reversible, but to synthesise glycogen, the substrate glucose-1-phosphate, phosphorylase and also the branching enzyme (Larner 1953), a transglucosidase, is required to form 1 : 6 linked glucose residues, because phosphorylase catalyses only the formation of 1 : 4 glucosidic linkages.

Glycogen synthetase, the enzyme forming glycogen from uridyldiphosphate-glucose also exists in two forms. The activator-independent form (I or *a* form) is favoured at low glycogen concentrations and is activated by insulin and inorganic phosphates. The activator-dependent (D or *b* form) enzyme requires high glucose-6-phosphate concentrations as activator and is in-

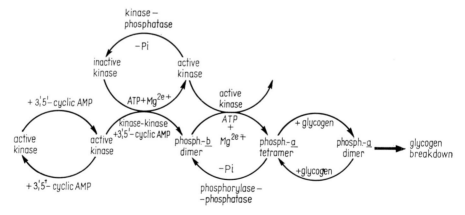

Figure 3.1. Activation of muscle glycogen phosphorylase according to Helmreich
(1970)

hibited by phosphates. The I form is transformed to D in the presence of ATP and Mg^{2+}, thus in the case of glycogen, synthetase D is the phosphorylated form. Cyclic AMP stimulates the actiivity of protein kinase which in turn transforms the I form into the D form. The reverse transformation (D to I) is catalysed by a phosphatase (Yip and Larner 1969, Villar-Palasi et al. 1970) (Figure 3.1).

The phosphorylase activity was found by several authors to be reduced in many tumour tissues. Decreased activities were found in ascites tumour cells (Nirenberg 1959), mammary and uterus carcinomas (Godlewski 1963) and in ascites and cancer cells (Sakeuchi and Ohama 1958).

Racker et. al. (1960) established the prevalence of the less active b phosphorylase in HeLa tumour cells. The phospsorylase and braching enzyme activity was relatively high in the more differentiated brain tumours (astrocytoma, meningioma) than in the more malignant type (medulloblastoma, spongioblastoma). Histochemical methods revealed that reactive cells possess a high activity which is not only in hypertrophic and gemistocytic astrocytes, but also in giant cells and perivascular tissue. The phosphorylase activity present in brain tumour cells is also mainly in the inactive b form. For full activity it was necessary to transform it into the active a form. (Viale and Ibba 1964).

Essentially the same is valid for glycogen synthetase (UDP glucose transferase). An invariably low activity has been found in hepatomas, sarcomas and HeLa cells (Racker et al. 1960., Nigam et al. 1962). In brain tumours the activity is similarly reduced in the more differentiated hypertrophic and reactive cells, as with phosphorylase in neuroectodermal tumours (Ibba and Viale 1964). According to Nasu (1964) all enzymes in gliomas responsible for glycogen breakdown and synthesis are located in the cell plasma.

2. Hexosephosphate metabolism

The glucose-1-phosphate produced by phosphorylase is transformed by phosphoglucomutase to glucose-6-phosphate. The cofactors of the enzyme activity are glucose-1-diphosphate and Mg^{2+}. The equilibrium of the reaction is on the glucose-6-phosphate side (95%).

The enzyme is present in cerebral cortex at a considerably higher level than in neuroectodermal tumours as measured by quantitative microchemical methods (Viale and Ibba 1964). Relatively high activities were found in astrocytomas and low activities in medulloblastomas, glioblastomas and spongioblastomas. Activities in ependymomas and meningiomas were higher than in normal frontal cortex. According to Lehrer (1962) the phosphoglucomutase activity in glial tumours was average to high, showing no consistent trend. Spencer et al. (1964) reported three distinct genetically determined patterns of phosphoglucomutase isoenzymes in human haemolysates. Data on brain and brain tumour isoenzymes are still lacking.

If glucose is directly accessible, glycolysis starts by phosphorylating glucose to glucose-6-phosphate with the aid of hexokinase, ATP and Mg^{2+}.

Glucose is the major substrate for glycolytic mechanisms and thus hexo-kinase must play a rôle in all aspects of glucose metabolism.

The characteristic features of brain hexokinase are its particulate nature, 85–90% in the bound form in contrast to 35–75% in other tissue (Crane and Sols 1953) and its relatively similar affinity for glucose and mannose and decreased affinity for fructose. This makes the hexokinase of nervous tissue in some respects similar to that of tumours (Wu and Racker 1959, Yushok 1959). Another peculiarity of brain hexokinase in contrast to yeast hexo-kinase is its non-competitive allosteric product (glucose-6-phosphate) in-hibition. ADP inhibits by competition with APT. Thus brain hexokinase is regulated by hexose-6-phosphate and ADP levels. Increased production of hexose-6-phosphate leads to complete inhibition mainly using the soluble brain hexokinase (Tuttle and Wilson 1970). Whether the tumour hexokinase possesses the same qualities is not yet clear.

The activity of hexokinase in tumour tissue is quite high. Ács et al. (1955) found in Ehrlich ascites tumour mitochondria a higher activity than in normal brain or liver. The level of hexokinase was found to parallel the tumour growth in several cases (MacNair et al. 1960, 1962; Lange and Kohn 1961).

In most brain tumours (twelve gliomas) Lehrer (1962) reported relatively low values of hexokinase activity. Perria et al. (1964) encountered high levels of hexokinase activity in the less differentiated tumours, such as medullo-blastoma and glioblastoma, and even higher activities in endothelial menin-giomas, compared with normal frontal cortex.

Most authors conclude that hexokinase activity is lower in the more differentiated gliomas and higher in atypical immature tumours.

Glucose-6-phosphatase is present in adult liver, kidney and brain micro-somes in decreasing order and absent or very low in lung, muscle, embryonic liver and several tumours (Weber and Cantero 1955, 1957). Glucose-6-phosphatase catalyses the reverse reaction of hexokinase, that is, it splits glucose-6-phosphate into glucose and inorganic phosphate. It is almost totally absent from malignant brain tumours and is only present in the more differentiated cells (Perria et al. 1964). It can be speculated that the absence of glucose-6-phosphatase from tumours conserves glucose-6-phos-phate which may be used for energy production in glycolysis or in the pen-tose phosphate pathway for the synthesis of ribose (Weber and Morris 1963).

Before dealing with the next enzyme in glycolysis a few words must be said about fructose phosphorylation in brain. The utilisation of fructose by brain in vivo is very low (Klein et al. 1947, Geiger et al. 1954) although in vitro it is capable of rapid oxidation similar to glucose (Wenner and Wein-house 1953, Meyerhof and Geliazkova 1947, Meyerhof and Wilson 1948). Because brain tissue lacks specific fructokinase activity, hexokinase con-verts fructose to fructose-6-phosphate as already noted; but as fructose has a lower affinity for the enzyme, it is utilised less under anaerobic conditions where ATP is rate limiting. In aerobic glycolysis, where ATP is not a limiting factor, fructose may also serve as substrate.

Tumour tissue is capable of various degrees of fructolysis. 15–50% of the oxygen uptake with glucose has been reported with fructose (Aisenberg

1961), thus it may represent an additional pathway essential for energy production in rapidly growing neoplastic tissue.

Phosphohexoisomerase is involved in the conversion of glucose-6-phosphate to fructose-6-phosphate. Phosphohexoisomerase activity is high in cerebral tissue; in fact this activity is higher in nerve cells than in oligodendroglia (Davison 1965) and five times higher in the glial cells per unit volume (Lowry *et al.* 1956). Warburg and Christian (1942) noticed elevated activities in tumours. Bodansky (1954, 1956) measured phosphohexoisomerase activities in sera of patients with metastatic carcinoma and found a correlation between the enzyme activity and the degree of metastasis. Viale and Ibba (1964) reported that high phosphohexoisomerase activity is characteristic of atypical tumour cells, thus the more differentiated astrocytomas reveal a lower activity compared with the less differentiated atypical astrocytomas and the polymorphous zone of glioblastoma. However, the highest activity was displayed by ependymomas. Comparing the phosphohexoisomerase activity of astrocytomas with normal astrocytes, Paxton (1959) found higher values in the tumours. Buckell and Robertson (1965) found high activities in the serum, CSF, and cystic fluids in glioma and cerebral metastatic carcinoma bearing patients. De Risio and Cumings (1960), Bruns *et al.* (1956) and Thompson (1959) also reported high phosphohexoisomerase activities in the CSF of brain tumour bearing patients.

The high glycolytic activity of malignant tumours is emphasised even more by the elevated levels of phosphofructokinase activity. This enzyme catalyses the transformation of fructose-6-phosphate into fructose-1,6-diphosphate in the presence of ATP and Mg^{2+}.

Phosphofructokinase, like phosphorylase, is activated by cyclic AMP (Mansour 1966) and inhibited by citrate or an excess of ATP (Lowry and Passoneau 1962). Cerebral tissue possesses relatively high activities. The phosphofructokinase activity of tumours is similar to hexokinase activity in requiring one molecule of ATP for one molecule of substrate. According to Viale and Ibba (1964) every investigated brain tumour revealed higher phosphofructokinase activity than normal cerebral frontal cortex. Glioblastoma, medulloblastoma and atypical astrocytoma were among the highest in addition to meningioma. Atypical tumour cells in the gliomas displayed highest activities.

The last enzyme in the anaerobic hexose phosphate metabolism is aldolase, previously called zymohexase because of its hexose-splitting rôle in fermentation. Aldolase converts fructose-1,6-diphosphate into 3-phosphoglyceraldehyde and dihydroxyacetone phosphate. After skeletal muscle, brain tissue has the highest aldolase activity among animal tissues (Sibley and Lehninger 1949).

Aldolase activity was found to be uniformly distributed in the different layers of Ammon's horn of rabbit and in the cerebral cortex of monkey; however, higher levels have been found in monkey cerebellar cortex (Robins *et al.* 1957, Lowry *et al.* 1954). Using fructose-1,6-diphosphate or fructose-1-phosphate as substrate, differences in muscle, liver and brain tissue aldolase have been recognised. Thus liver aldolase uses both in an equal ratio and skeletal muscle tissue aldolase acts primarily on fructose-1,6-diphosphate and slightly on fructose-1-phosphate. Brain tissue aldolase activity ratio, that is the activity with fructose-1,6-diphosphate divided by the activity with fructose-1-phosphate is around ten in contrast to fifty in muscle and one in liver. Competitive inhibition of muscle aldolase with ATP also differentiates it from liver aldolase, which is not inhibited by ATP (Spolter et al. 1965).

The reason for this selective behaviour toward the two substrates was better understood when the different molecular forms of enzymes were demonstrated. Using gel electrophoretic methods three distinct forms could be revealed and also several hybrids. The 'a' form (muscle) migrated next to the cathode, the 'c' form (brain) to the anode and the 'b' form (liver) was between the two of them (Penhoet et al. 1966). The pattern was shown to change during development; for example, foetal liver had an a pattern (Shapira et al. 1968; Hers and Joassin 1961). Transformation of aldolase-types not only occurred during embryonic development but also in pathological cases, primarily in oncogenesis.

Based on quantitative measurements of aldolase activity, Warburg and Christian (1942) found that the elevation of serum aldolase in sarcomas was first detectable when the tumour reached a size greater than 2–3% of the body weight. If the tumour was excised or its growth inhibited, the elevated aldolase activity declined to a normal value. Extending the measurements to man they found in about 20% of one hundred and four cases of cancer an elevated level of serum aldolase. The investigations of Warburg and Hiepler (1952), Sibley et al. (1955), Sibley (1958) and Wu (1959) on the release of aldolase in Ehrlich ascites cells led to the conclusion that anaerobic incubation and the absence of glucose or the addition of dinitrophenol increased the differential loss of some ascites cell enzymes.

Perria et al. (1964) reported higher aldolase activities in meningiomas, ependimomas and glioblastomas. There was again a tendency in the atypical gliomas towards higher levels of aldolase activity. There seemed to be an inverse relationship between the aldolase activity and the hexosemono-phosphate oxidative pathway enzymes in the tumours. High aldolase activities paralleled low glucose-6-phosphate dehydrogenase activities.

With the development of molecular enzymology and research on protein structure, new diagnostic and therapeutic possibilities appeared in tumour chemistry. The demonstration of isoenzymes, that is, tissue and species-specific multiple molecular forms of enzymes, is one of the major accomplishments of molecular enzymology. Aldolase exists in the form of iso-enzymes with four subunits and appears, as already mentioned, in three basic forms. Rutter et al. (1963) and Shapira et al. (1968) first observed that aldolase of liver hepatoma was present not in the b but in the a form. In molecular diseases, however, the c type is increased and the a type decreased. Sugimura et al. (1970) also found aldolase a and c in Yoshida ascites hepatomas. The aldolase in Novikoff hepatoma was identified as normal muscle aldolase a by several criteria (Brox et al. 1969). In slowly growing hepatomas, aldolase a and b and their hybrids were observed by Matsushima et al. (1968). This means that the liver aldolase was still retained in the well differentiated hepatomas, but was largely or completely replaced by the muscle type aldolase in the poorly differentiated tumours.

According to Sugimura *et al.* (1969) the normal human cerebral cortex showed bands of aldolase *a* and *c* and three hybrid bands. The pattern was the same in white matter. Glioblastoma also possessed aldolase *a* and *c* and their hybrids, but meningioma lacked aldolase *c* and showed only aldolase *a* activity. This difference in aldolase isoenzymes is also reflected in substrate specificity. Cerebral cortex had a ration of fructose-1,6-diphosphate/fructose-1-phosphate equal to 19.2; glioblastoma 28.8 and meningioma 47.6. Our own experiments on isoenzymes of tumour aldolase and foetal brain aldolase also revealed a change from the *c* type towards the *a* type (Figures 1.3, 3.2).

A common feature of the tumour aldolase type modifications is their 'foetal-like' pattern, which is an expression of the molecular dedifferentiation characterised by the repression of the synthesis of the tissue specific forms of enzymes (Herskovitz *et al.* 1967). It will be seen later that this occurs with other enzymes, and is therefore a general phenomenon (Figure 3.3).

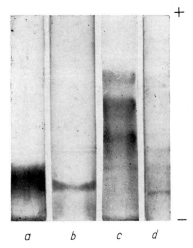

Figure 3.2. Aldolase isoenzymes crystallised from rabbit muscle (*a*), glioblastoma multiforme No. 288 (*b*), mixed glioma No. 319 (*c*) and glioblastoma multiforme No. 258 (*d*)

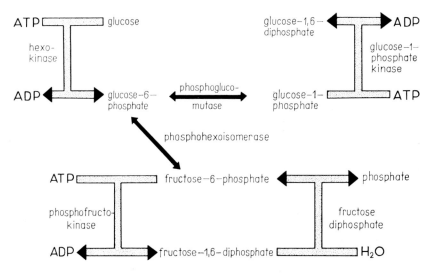

Figure 3.3. Metabolism of hexosephosphates

4*

3. Triosephosphate metabolism

Dihydroxyacetone phosphate formed by aldolase is converted into 3-phosphoglyceraldehyde by phosphotriose isomerase. Studies of this enzyme have not been conducted in brain tumours. Glycolytic triosephosphate metabolism proceeds with the conversion of 3-phosphoglyceraldehyde, which is dehydrogenated and phosphorylated by phosphoglyceraldehyde dehydrogenase. This is another 'key' enzyme in glycolysis. It transforms glyceraldehyde-3-phosphate into 1,3-diphosphoglyceric acid. The enzyme requires NAD and inorganic phosphate for activity. It is built from four subunits similar to aldolase and lactic dehydrogenase. One molecule of coenzyme is firmly bound to each subunit. Each subunit contains a reactive SH group in position 149 and a reactive lysine in position 183 for the binding of the coenzyme and of the substrate (Harris and Perham 1968, Polgár 1964). Blocking the SH group with iodoacetic acid or p-chloromercuribenzoate stopped the enzyme activity (Harris et al. 1963). Brain phosphoglyceraldehyde dehydrogenase is particularly sensitive to iodoacetate (Himwich 1951). The enzymic reaction proceeds in at least two steps, first dehydrogenation and then phosphorylation (Velick and Hayes 1953).

Diphosphoglycerate phosphokinase catalyses the first ATP generating step in glycolysis, converting 1,3-diphosphoglycerate in the presence of ADP as phosphate acceptor into 3-phosphoglycerate and ATP.

In spite of the importance of phosphoglyceraldehyde dehydrogenase and diphosphoglycerate phosphokinase in glycolysis, there are few studies of their general oncology and their relationship to brain tumours. Perria et al. (1964) revealed highest enzyme activities in glioblastomas and meningiomas and lowest activities in typical astrocytomas; all specimens investigated except astrocytomas had higher activities than normal frontal cortex. High activities were apparent in all kinds of undifferentiated and atypical neoplastic cells.

In the next metabolic step 3-phosphoglycerate is converted first by a phosphoglyceromutase to 2-phosphoglycerate, which is in turn dehydrogenated by enolase to phosphoenolpyruvate. Enolase is inhibited by fluoride, which binds the Mg^{2+} necessary for enzyme activity. Phosphoenolpyruvate is a molecule with an energy-rich phosphate bond capable of yielding ATP. Thus in the presence of phosphoenolpyruvate phosphokinase and ADP as phosphate acceptor, ATP is synthesised from phosphoenolpyruvate; this is the second molecule of ATP formed during the glycolytic cycle. The latter enzyme was studied by Lehrer (1962) in gliomas and found to be present at relatively normal levels in most tumours.

4. Lactic acid dehydrogenase

Lactic acid dehydrogenase (LDH) has been the subject of most investigations into tumour metabolism since Warburg published his results on the increased anaerobic glycolysis of tumours in 1930.

The quantitative method for lactate dehydrogenase activity measurement now widely used in all NADH-linked enzyme activity determinations,

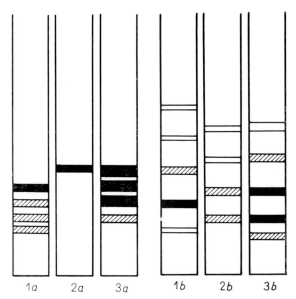

Figure 3.4. LDH isoenzymes from tumour surrounding tissue (*a*) and tumour (*b*) of glioblastoma No.
33; nuclear (1), mitochondrial (2) and supernatant
(3) cell fractions

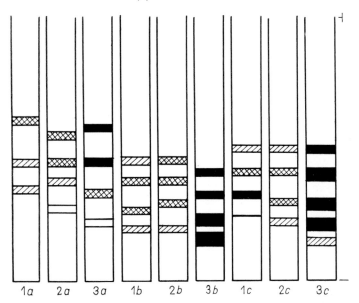

Figure 3.5. LDH isoenzymes from cell fractions of human temporal lobe (*a*), tumour surrounding tissue (*b*) and tumour (*c*) of
spongioblastoma No. 105; nuclear (1), mitochondrial (2) and
supernatant (3) cell fractions

was described by Kubowitz and Ott in 1943. They also succeeded in the
isolation of LDH from tumours. These investigations were extended later
to the measurement of lactate dehydrogenase in serum and CSF, which
was found to be elevated in neoplastic, inflammatory and degenerative
diseases (Hill and Levi 1954, Wróblewski and LaDue 1955, Wróblewski
and Decker 1957, Bruns et al. 1956, Fleischer et al. 1957, Green et al.
1958).

In transplanted tumours, lactate dehydrogenase increased promptly and
continued to increase until death; in cases of tumour regression it decreased
(Hsieh et al. 1955, 1959, Friend and Wróblewski 1956, Hill and Jordan,
1957, Mango et al. 1958). According to Hsieh et al. (1959) the elevated lactate
dehydrogenase levels did not disappear as consistently as increased aldolase
levels after excision of the tumours. Thus it could not be simply the result
of enzyme leakage but was rather an enzyme inducing effect of the tumour
cells in the organism of the host. This effect very much resembles the mechanism of enzyme induction in virus infections. Wróblewski (1958) concluded also that the rise in LDH levels was due to release of the enzyme by
the tumour or liver.

The diagnostic value of lactate dehydrogenase determinations on body
fluids is diminished by the relative nonspecificity of the reaction already
mentioned. High levels of lactate dehydrogenase were encountered by
Corridori et al. (1960) in investigations of brain tumours and more noticeably
in malignant neoplasms. The activity of lactic acid dehydrogenase in the
CSF was not related to the histological type of tumour. According to Lehrer
(1962), the lactate level was also increased in malignant tumours.

Kirsch (1969) found that in experimental glioblastomas there was a
higher lactate production in the periphery of the tumours in comparison
to the tumour core. In our own investigations (Wollemann et al. 1969)
a high lactate dehydrogenase activity was also localised in the surrounding
tissue of tumours (Figures 3.4, 3.5).

The lactic acid dehydrogenase activity was not consistently elevated in
all brain tumours or serum. Increased levels were observed in about 30%
of all cases and in 50% of cases in the CSF (De Risio and Cumings 1960,
Fleischer et al. 1957). LDH activity measurements were also performed in
cystic fluids (Buckell and Robertson 1965, Szliwovski and Cumings 1961),
where consistently increased levels were observed in all cases. With microchemical methods high activity levels of lactate dehydrogenase were found
in medulloblastoma, glioblastoma, atypical astrocytoma and oligodendroglioma. Among benign tumours, neurinoma, meningioma and ependymoma
also showed high activities (Perria et al. 1964). After these results became
well known and histochemical methods for NAD and NADH linked dehydrogenase activities became available, subsequent studies showed lactate
dehydrogenase activity in tumour cells. High activities were localised in
the reactive, hypertrophic and gemistocytic astrocytes in the giant cells of
glioblastoma and sarcoma and in the areas of vascular endothelial proliferation (Andreussi and Restelli-Fondelli 1966, Rubinstein and Sutton 1964).
However, Chason et al. (1963) stated that the activity of neoplastic cells in
tumours was relatively higher than the activity of the reactive cells.

In our own investigations (Wollemann *et al*. 1965, 1969, Wollemann 1967, 1970) LDH activity was demonstrated in tissue slides and stained after the method of Hess *et al*. (1958) in human brain tumours and experimentally induced or transplanted brain tumours in mice. In histochemical sections, LDH activity was intense not only in astrocytes of gemistocytic tumours but also in the areas of vascular endothelial proliferation. Intense lactate dehydrogenase activity was observed both in benign and malignant astro-

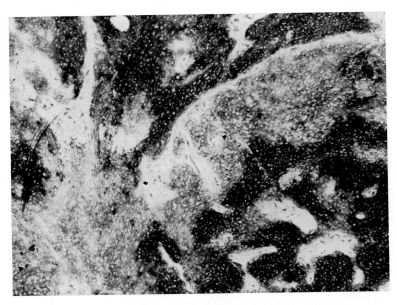

Figure 3.6. LDH activity of endotheliomatous meningioma No. 193. Histochemical slide stained for LDH activity according to Hess *et al*. (1958). Typical marmorate pattern of enzyme activity in which areas of strong activity are contiguous with zones of low or moderate activity. Little enzyme activity is present in the connective tissue stroma or blood vessel walls. Magnification 82 ×

cytomas and also in glioblastoma multiforme; the astrocytic tumour cells showed considerable oxidative enzyme activity. Wherever necrosis was present within the tumour, the enzymic reaction was invariably negative. In the neurinomas, the cells of the Antoni-B type demonstrated intensive LDH activity. In metastatic carcinomas and experimentally induced tumours, intense histochemical reactions were observed in tumour cells where necrotic areas were absent. A high activity was present in the reactive astrocytes of the adjacent oedematous brain areas. The reactive glial cells usually showed a stronger histochemical reaction than the anaplastic tumour cells (Figures 3.6, 3.7).

Tissue cultures of brain tumours revealed elevated activities similar to those of the original tumour (Figures 3.8, 3.9). Variability in the polymorphous glioblastomas and giant cell sarcomas persisted in the cultivated tumour cells which, according to Kreuzberg *et al.* (1966), demonstrates a general disorder of enzyme production. Data on the increase of different dehydrogenase activities in tissue cultures in brain tumours are also reported by Matakas (1969).

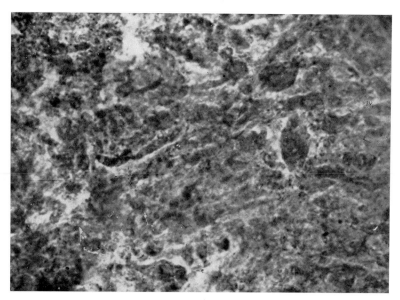

Figure 3.7. LDH activity of experimentally induced glioma in mice by the method of Zimmermann and Arnold (1941). Intensive LDH activity in the tumour cells revealed by the histochemical method of Hess *et al.* (1958). Cell nuclei are not stained. Magnification 160 ×

Lactic acid dehydrogenase was the first enzyme to be recognised as existing in multiple molecular forms, that is, as isoenzymes. This was discovered independently by three groups in 1957 (Vessel and Bearn, Wieland and Pfleiderer, Sayde and Hill) although Emil Fischer in 1895 reported the presence of enzymes in different species or organs catalysing the same reaction but differing in their structure. Evidence that aldolase from yeast differed from that of animal tissue was reported by Warburg and Christian (1942); additional data have become available concerning isoenzyme patterns of digestive enzymes from various sources. These earlier investigations, however, differed from those performed at the end of the 1950's. The later work demonstrated that the four subunits which form one molecule of LDH may consist of two kinds of polypeptides, named H and M after their occurrence in heart and skeletal muscle. Pure H_4 can be crystallised from heart and M_4 from muscle. LDH separated from different organs by gel electrophoresis may appear in five bands moving from cathode to anode: M_4 (LDH$_5$), HM$_3$, (LDH$_4$), H_2M_2 (LDH$_3$), H_3M (LDH$_2$) and H_4 (LDH$_1$). LDH$_2$, LDH$_3$ and LDH$_4$ are hybrids, LDH$_1$ and LDH$_5$ are pure isoenzymes.

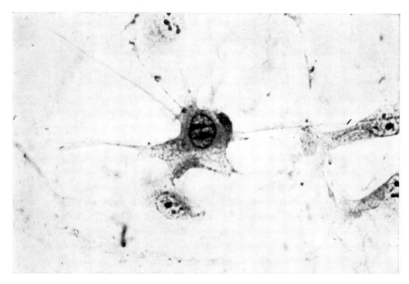

Figure 3.8. LDH activity of a tissue culture of endotheliomatous meningioma No. 144. In the centre, strong activity in one arachnoidal cell; epithelial cells show less activity. Tissue culture twelve days old. Magnification 500 ×

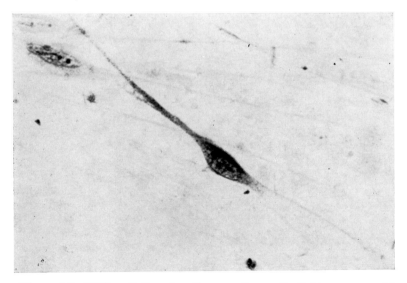

Figure 3.9. LDH activity of a tissue culture of glioblastoma multiforme No. 149. Strong LDH activity in a piloid astrocyte in the centre, surrounded by other tumour cells showing no activity. Magnification 500 ×

The isoenzyme name was proposed by Markert and Moller (1959) who first stained isoenzymes on gels with the method essentially employed in histochemistry. Later, Wieland and Pfleiderer (1962) proposed the name 'isoenzyme' for those enzymes which are derived from the same organ or tissue and have the same catalytic action. They called 'heteroenzymes' those enzymes which have the same catalytic action but are derived from different organs or even from different species. Generally, molecular weight differences between heteroenzymes are more pronounced than those between isoenzymes. Differences in the distribution of isoenzymes may occur within the same cell between the mitochondrial and plasmal enzymes, as for example in the case of malate dehydrogenase (Grimm and Doherty 1961), and lactate dehydrogenase (Agostini et al. 1966, Güttler 1967).

Diagnostic methods based on the specificity of the lactate dehydrogenase increase in serum, CSF, malignant effusions and cystic fluids were further elaborated when the separation of LDH isoenzymes became known. The increased lactate dehydrogenase activity caused by cardiac or cerebral infarctions could be sharply differentiated from the neoplastic enhancement of lactate dehydrogenase activity. Vascular lesions increased the activity of LDH_1 in the serum, whereas neoplastic diseases increased the activity of LDH_3, LDH_4 or LDH_5, depending on the kind of tumour (Wróblewski and Gregory 1961). LDH_1 prevails in normal brain tissue and CSF and LDH_2 in normal serum; thus the possibility exists for determining the origin of increased LDH activities in these fluids and tissues. Inflammatory diseases

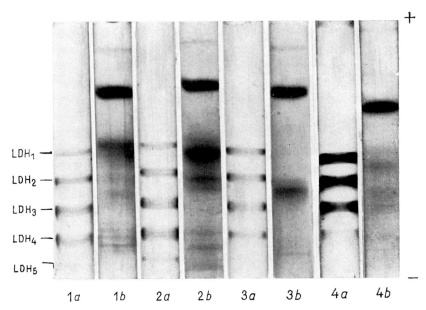

Figure 3.10. LDH isoenzyme (a) and protein (b) patterns of glioblastoma multiforme No. 79 (1), meningioma endothel. No. 80 (2), malignant astrocytoma. No. 81 (3) and fibrillar astrocytoma No. 4 (4)

present a complication to diagnosis since LDH_3 isoenzyme is also increased in these cases. In the glioma group a parallelism was found between the mobility of LDH isoenzymes and malignity. The more malignant glioblastomas revealed higher LDH_4 and LDH_5 activities and at times, double bands also appeared (Gerhardt *et al.* 1963, Wollemann *et al.* 1965). In more benign astrocytomas and oligodendrogliomas LDH_2 and LDH_3 display the strongest activity (Figure 3.10, Table IV).

TABLE IV

Distribution of lactate dehydrogenase activity
in human brain tumours on starch gel electrophoresis
(Figures represent percentage contribution
of each band to the total activity)

Tumour No.	Band No.				
	LDH_1	LDH_2	LDH_3	LDH_4	LDH_5
Glioblastoma					
No. 174	18	29	30	23	—
No. 48	22	46	23	9	—
No. 195	14	23	34	29	—
No. 411	11	17	38	21	13
Oligodendroglioma					
No. 257	60	23	17	—	—
No. 350	40	39	21	—	—
Astrocytoma					
No. 160	20	24	35	21	—
No. 126	35	31	34	—	—
Meningioma (end.)					
No. 193	2	5	20	34	41
No. 432	17	14	41	28	—
No. 440	11	20	32	25	12
No. 197	14	26	36	24	—
No. 348	7	17	30	46	—
Meningioma (fibr.)					
No. 166	10	18	42	30	—
Metastic carcinoma					
No. 164	26	34	40	—	—
No. 167	7	11	29	53	—
No. 90	15	36	28	21	—
Neuroblastoma					
No. 132	20	32	25	23	—

Bonavita and Guarneri (1963) observed no differences between the LDH pattern of white and grey matter in the same lobe of ox brain. Hence, it can be concluded that differences in the LDH patterns in oligodendrogliomas or astrocytomas cannot be ascribed to the presence of normal glial cells or the lack of neurones, but rather to the degree of malignity. Similar results were obtained by Sano *et al.* (1966) and Shervin *et al.* (1968). Increased LDH activity and the tumour-like LDH pattern were generally present in tissue surrounding brain tumours in adults and infants (Wollemann *et al.* 1969). As to the origin of the altered LDH pattern in the tumour surrounding tissue, Langvad (1968) has concluded on the basis of studies with colonic tumours that anatomical changes occur later than the enzymatic transformation. The differences in LDH activity between the cell fractions of tumours and tissue surrounding the tumour were not significant in the supernatant fraction, although the particulate cell fractions revealed significantly higher LDH activities in the mitochondrial and nuclear cell fractions of tumours (Table V). The LDH isoenzyme pattern in the particulate frac-

TABLE V

*LDH activity in µM/0.1 ml/min in tumour
and control brain cell fractions (Nagy et. al 1971)*

	Nuclei	Mitochondria	Supernatant
Tumours	8.5±0.8	9.0±1.2	49.5±3.6
Control	5.1±0.4	5.1±0.4	41.5±2.1

tions of tumours was also changed, though to a lesser degree than that of the supernatant. The LDH pattern of tissue surrounding the tumour was changed only in the supernatant fraction (Figures 3.4, 3.5).

Essentially similar changes of LDH pattern in malignancy (Figure 3.11 *a*, *b*) and in histochemical slides of brain tumours (Figure 3.7) were also obtained by our group (Katona *et al.* 1965) in experimentally induced and transplanted brain tumours in mice produced by methylcholanthrene implantation (Zimmermann and Arnold 1941). Dawson *et al.* (1964) concluded that the rate of synthesis of the two major forms of lactic dehydrogenase can be correlated with metabolic differentiation. Aeration with gas mixtures containing less than 20% oxygen resulted in a relative increase of the isoenzymes rich in M subunits, whereas higher oxygen concentrations increased the H containing isoenzymes in tissue cultures of human lymphocytes (Hellung-Larsen and Andersen 1970). Güttler and Clausen (1969) concluded from cultured kidney cortex cells that apart from the oxygen supply, the rate of glycolysis and cell division also influenced the LDH pattern. Our results obtained in tissue cultures of benign and malignant human brain tumours (Wollemann *et al.* 1972) established that although the LDH pattern changed generally to the M type, there were individual differences even under similar oxygen supply conditions, that is, tumours having originally similar LDH patterns, may differ significantly after being grown in tissue culture, according to the cell type which has been enriched during cultivation (Figures 3.10, 3.12) (Wollemann *et al.* 1971). Among benign brain tumours, neurinomas and endothelial meningiomas also reveal M type LDH patterns (Gerhardt *et al.* 1963, Wollemann *et al.* 1965), perhaps because normal connective tissue and peripheral nervous tissue have similar patterns (Lowenthal *et al.* 1964, Gerhardt *et al.* 1963).

The serum and CSF lactate dehydrogenase activities and isoenzymes, contrary to the report of Green *et al.* (1958), are not always changed, because normal LDH levels occur in 50–70% of the cases (De Risio and Cumings 1960, Fleischer *et al.* 1957, Wollemann *et al.* 1960). However, the lactate

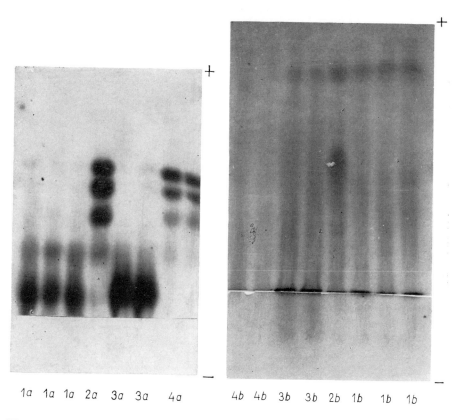

1a 1a 1a 2a 3a 3a 4a 4b 4b 3b 3b 2b 1b 1b 1b

Figure 3.11. LDH isoenzyme (*a*) and protein patterns (*b*) demonstrated on a starch gel electrophorogram of experimentally induced gliomas in mice (1), heart (2) muscle (3) and brain (4) from normal mice supernatants of homogenates

dehydrogenase activity and the pattern in cystic fluids of brain tumours always changed in parallel with malignancy and differed sharply from the normal serum LDH pattern (Szliwovski and Cumings 1961, Wollemann *et al.* 1969).

However, in cases of encapsulated hygromas and cystic craniopharyngeomas (Wollemann *et al.* 1969) the M type LDH subunits also prevailed (Figures 3.13, 3.14). (In the former case the connective tissue of the capsule might be the cause of M type LDH, in the latter the rapid release pointed to the relative malignancy of the tumour.

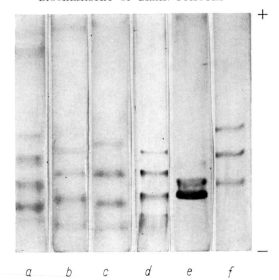

Figure 3.12. LDH isoenzymes from tissue cultures of glioblastoma multiforme No. 79 (*a*); meningioma endothel. No. 80 (*b*); astrocytoma malign. No. 81 (*c*); astrocytoma fibrillare No. 54 (*d*); glioblastoma multiforme No. 258 (*e*); meningioma endothel. No. 261 (*f*)

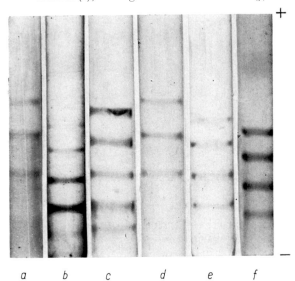

Figure 3.13. LDH isoenzymes from serum (*a*) and cyst (*b*) of glioblastoma multiforme No. 114, tumour (*c*) and CSF (*d*) from medulloblastoma No. 279, cystic fluid from mixed glioma No. 319 (*e*), and from oligodendroglioma No. 265 (*f*)

As in the case of aldolase, the LDH pattern of foetal tissue very much resembles that of tumours, thus in both cases of rapid cell growth the more primitive pattern of enzyme structure reappears (Gerhardt *et al.* 1963, Wollemann *et al.* 1971) (Figures 3.15, 3.16).

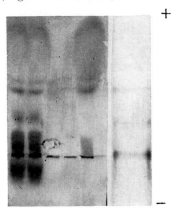

1a 1a 1b 1b 1c   2d

Figure 3.14. LDH isoenzymes from cystic fluids (*a, d*), CSF (*b*) and serum (*c*) from craniopharyngeoma No. 23 demonstrated by starch gel (1) and disc gel (2) electro- phoresis

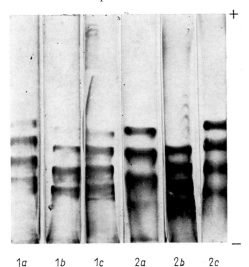

1a   1b   1c   2a   2b   2c

Figure 3.15. LDH isoenzymes from dif- ferent parts of twenty (1) and twenty- eight (2) weeks old human embryonic brain: frontal cortex (*a*), white matter (*b*) and mesencephalon (*c*)

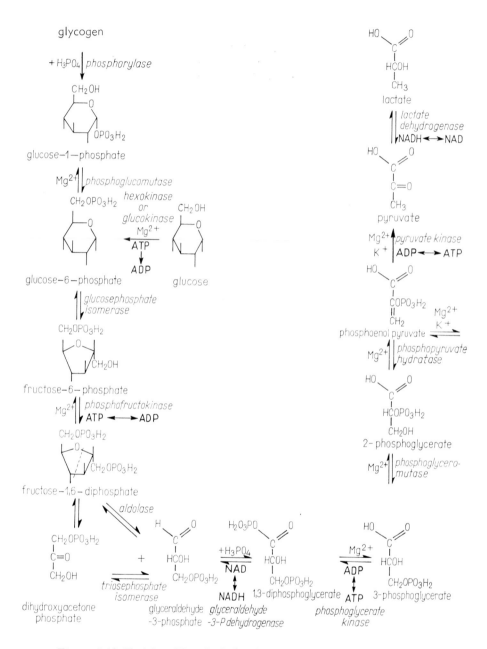

Figure 3.16. Embden–Meyerhof glycolytic pathway (Falconer 1969)

5. *Alcohol dehydrogenase*

Alcohol dehydrogenase, like lactic dehydrogenase, is a NADH dependent dehydrogenase. It participates in yeast glycolysis but not in the glycolytic pathway in animal cells; in liver this enzyme consists of two subunits since it has a dimeric structure (Pietruczko and Theorell 1969). One of the two forms uses ethanol as substrate, the other steroids and the hybrid forms use both substrates. Liver alcohol dehydrogenase is localised in the soluble part of the cytoplasm. The occurrence of alcohol dehydrogenase in normal brain had been denied by several authors (Beer and Quastel 1958, Towne 1964, Räihä and Koskinen 1964) until recently, when more sensitive methods were used and Raskin and Sokoloff (1968) stated that the alcohol dehydrogenase activity of brain was about a thousand times less than the activity of liver. The kinetic properties of the brain enzyme and responses to inhibitors were similar to the liver enzyme. The authors assume that a cerebral enzymic mechanism which oxidises ethanol may play a significant rôle in local regulations during exposure to ethanol and in the pathogenesis of the neural disorders associated with chronic alcohol ingestion or withdrawal. However a rôle in steroid and drug oxidation has also to be considered. Brain tumours showed a very slight activity. A few reports have been published on the remarkable activity of astrocytic cells in spongioblastomas (Nasu and Viale 1962), and higher activity during tissue culture in some cells of cerebellar astrocytoma document an increased activity (Gluszcz and Giernat 1969); cultured giant cells of gliomas displayed very weak alcohol dehydrogenase activity (Gluszcz and Giernat 1970).

The appearance of the changed isoenzyme patterns in cystic fluids, tumours, CSF and sera might be helpful in the diagnosis of brain tumours and in the problem of tumour genesis.

The relative ease of demonstration of LDH isoenzymes in minute quantities of body fluids or tissue makes the isoenzyme demonstration one of the most promising fields of molecular pathology.

In recent review articles on isoenzymes, the appearance of new foetal-like isoenzymes in cancer and experimental tumours has been explained by the depression of genes controlling foetal proteins (Weinhouse 1971, Criss 1971, Farron *et al.* 1972).

3.3. HEXOSEMONOPHOSPHATE SHUNT
(PENTOSE PHOSPHATE PATHWAY)

Apart from glucose-6-phosphate isomerisation and phosphorylation, glucose-6-phosphate can be also directly oxidised in the presence of NADP and Mg^{2+} (Dickens and Glock 1951) and further transformed through several steps to ribose-5-phosphate. Two molecules of ribose-5-phosphate are transformed into triosephosphate and heptulosephosphate, which may yield tetrose phosphate and fructosephosphate and ultimately triosephosphate with regeneration of hexosephosphate (Horecker and Smyrniotis 1953, Racker 1954) (Figure 3.17).

5

Changes of Glycolysis in Brain Tumours

Enzyme activity	Type of brain tumour															
	MT	BT	GL	GB	AC	OG	EM	SB	MB	NN	MG	MC	SO	CP	EI	TS
Glycolysis	+[6,7]															
Phosphorylase					+[11]						+[11]					
Phosphogluco-mutase	+[9]		+[8] −[9]	+[9]	+[9]	+[9]					+[9]					
Hexokinase	+[9]	−[9]	−[8]	+[9]					−[9]		+[9]					
Glucose-6-phosphatase	−[9]	+[9]														
Phosphohexose-isomerase	+[9]		+[13] +[16] +[12] +[24]									+[12] +[16] +[24]				
Phosphofructo-kinase	+[9]		+[9]	+[9]							+[9]					
Aldolase	+[9]		+[7]	+[7]	−[9]						+[9]					
3-Phosphoglycer-aldehyde dehydrogenase				+[9]							+[5]					
Phosphoenol-pyruvate kinase																
Lactate de-hydrogenase	+[14-17]		±[8] +[19] +[13] +[17] +[20] +[25]	+[9] +[10] +[21] +[22] +[2] +[3] +[4]	+[9]	+[9]	+[9]	+[9]		+[9]	+[9] +[21] +[22] +[2] +[4]	+[5]	+[10] +[27]	+[4]	+[18]	+[1]
Alcohol de-hydrogenase					+[23]			+[26]								

+ = increase, − = decrease, ± = unchanged.

[1] Funagalli et al. (1965), [2] Gerhardt et al. (1963), [3] Wollemann et al. (1965), [4] Wollemann et al. (1969), [5] Wollemann (1970), [6] Victor and Wolf (1937), [7] Heller and Elliott (1955), [8] Lehrer (1962), [9] Perria et al. (1964), [10] Kreuzberg et al. (1966), [11] Viale and Ibba (1964), [12] Buckell and Robertson (1965), [13] De Risio and Cumings (1960), [14] Wróblewski and LaDue (1955), [15] Wróblewski and Decker (1957), [16] Bruns et al. (1956), [17] Fleischer et al. (1957), [18] Kirsch (1969), [19] Corridori et al. (1960), [20] Szliwowski and Cumings (1961), [21] Sano et al. (1966), [22] Shervin et al. (1968), [23] Gluszcz and Giernat (1969), [24] Thompson et al. (1959), [25] Lehrer (1962), [26] Nasu and Viale (1962), [27] Andreussi and Restelli-Fondelli (1966).

The reaction sequence involves several metabolically important compounds, especially the ribosephosphates, which are concerned with nucleotide synthesis. The direct oxidation of glucose is not associated with the production of high energy phosphates, thus the aim of the hexosemonophosphate shunt is primarily ribose phosphate production for nucleic acid synthesis and sedoheptulose production for tyrosine synthesis.

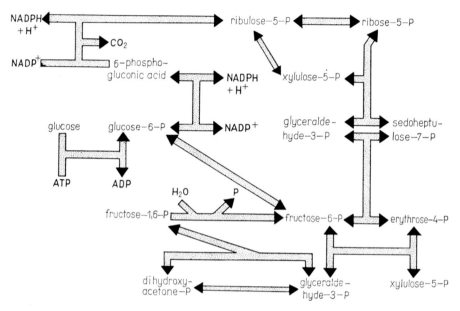

Figure 3.17. Hexosemonophosphate shunt

The pentose phosphate pathway is very active in liver, where about half of the metabolised glucose enters this cycle. In normal brain, although the enzymes of the hexosemonophosphate shunt are present, the low concentration of available NADP prevents it from functioning. In abnormal conditions, when the glycolytic pathway and tricarboxylic acid cycle are inhibited or are relatively insufficient, as in neoplastic disease, the activity of the pentose phosphate pathway rises considerably.

1. Levels of hexosemonophosphate shunt enzymes

The following two enzymes of the hexosemonophosphate shunt have been studied in detail in tumour metabolism: glucose-6-phosphate dehydrogenase and 6-phosphogluconate dehydrogenase.

Glucose-6-phosphate dehydrogenase was discovered first by Warburg and Christian (1931) in red blood cells and called *Zwischenferment*. Later it was shown to be present in a large series of normal and tumour tissues (Glock

5*

and McLean 1954). Highest activities were encountered in lactating mammary glands, adrenal glands, spleen and foetal tissues followed by the liver of rats. The enzyme levels in neoplasms were relatively high in tumours of lymphatic origin.

The isoenzymes of glucose-6-phosphate dehydrogenase were first recognised by Tsao (1960). Rat kidney and liver displayed three bands of enzyme activity and heart and erythrocytes two bands, but one band was detected in brain homogenate. In tissue cultures of mouse fibroblast cells and ascites lymphoma cells, the former appeared in two components, while the latter was homogeneous. Human cells from a culture of ovarian carcinoma exhibited two fast bands and one rather diffuse slower component.

Quantitative measurements of glucose-6-phosphate dehydrogenase activity were performed by several groups of authors on different brain tumours. Paxton (1959) revealed three to ten times higher activities in all investigated tumours irrespective of the histological type compared with the analogous normal tissue. Lehrer (1962a) showed average to high glucose-6-phosphate dehydrogenase activities in all investigated brain tumours, without a consistent trend. Perria *et al.* (1964) reported that in all investigated tumours except glioblastomas higher glucose-6-phosphate dehydrogenase activities

TABLE VI

Glucose-6-phosphate dehydrogenase activity* from supernatants of temqoral lobes and of brain tumours (A) and tissues surrounding brain tumours (B)

	Δ OD/mg protein	
	A	B
Astrocytoma		
No. 106	0.41	
No. 87	0.2	
Oligodendroglioma		
No. 123	0.54	
Spongioblastoma		
No. 38	0.2	0.1
No. 105	0.70	0.46
Ependymoma		
No. 84	0.59	
No. 195	0.61	
Meningioma (end.)		
No. 144	0.78	
Plexus papilloma		
No. 127	0.40	0.22
Temporal lobe		
No. 104	0.28	
No. 47	0.2	
No. 211	0.11	

*Glucose-6-phosphate dehydrogenase activity was measured according to Kornberg and Horecker (1953).

were encountered than in normal cerebral cortex. Among the tumours
spongioblastoma had the highest activity as demonstrated with chemical
methods. The latter authors concluded that increased or decreased activities
are not to be taken as a characteristic of atypical or cellular proliferation.
In our material (Wollemann *et al.* 1969) consisting of two astrocytomas,
two spongioblastomas, one oligodendroglioma, two ependymomas, one
meningioma and two plexus papillomas, all supernatants of tumour homogenates displayed higher activities than apparently normal grey and white
matter (Table VI). Gluszcz and Giernat (1969) concluded from tissue cultures

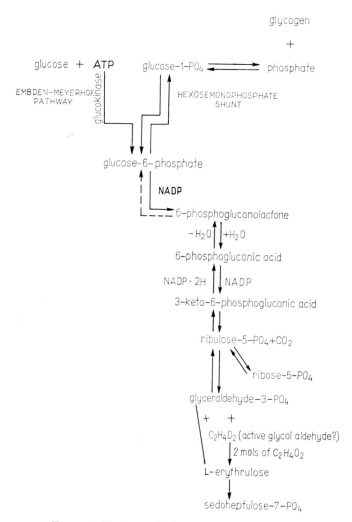

Figure 3.18. Interrelations of Embden–Meyerhof
pathway and hexosemonophosphate shunt

of gliomas, that among several oxidoreductases investigated the most ir-
regular activity in various cell populations was shown by glucose-6-phos-
phate dehydrogenase.

The second enzyme in the hexosemonophosphate shunt, 6-phosphoglu-
conate dehydrogenase was also investigated in brain tumours although to a
lesser degree. Its activity paralleled that of glucose-6-phosphate dehydrogenase according to Lehrer (1962) and Schiffer and Vesco (1962). Fildes and Parr
(1963) reported that 6-phosphogluconate dehydrogenase also occurs in two
genetically determined forms in human erythrocytes, thus research on
tumour material might also be useful.

From ^{14}C glucose experiments performed *in situ* by Sacks (1957) and from
work with human brain slices, Sutherland *et al.* (1955) concluded that the
Embden-Meyerhof glycolytic pathway (Fig. 3.16) is almost exclusively used
in human brain. Only during inhibition of this pathway, that is under abnormal conditions, was the hexosemonophosphate shunt active (Figure 3.18).
Similar investigations on patients with brain tumours would be of interest.
The reason for the apparent nonspecific increase of enzymes participating in
the hexosemonophosphate shunt in brain tumours could be the enhanced
demand of pentose phosphates for nucleic acid synthesis, that is cell replication. Similar changes also occur in embryonic tissue. Owing to the 2–5
fold increase in hexosemonophosphate shunt enzyme activities of glial
cells in comparison with nerve cells, the elevated activities in gliomas can
be considered also as glial activity (Davison 1965).

3.4. RESPIRATORY ENZYMES

1. Tricarboxylic acid cycle

Respiratory enzymes can be included in two main groups, the tricarboxylic
acid cycle and terminal respiration. The tricarboxylic acid cycle is also
called Krebs or Szentgyörgyi–Krebs cycle, because Szentgyörgyi first
observed that some organic dicarboxylic acids, such as succinic, fumaric
and oxaloacetic catalytically increased pyruvate oxidation whereas malonic
acid inhibited it. The reaction mechanism was elucidated by Krebs, who
demonstrated citrate synthesis by the condensation of pyruvic acid and
oxaloacetic acid with carbon dioxide liberation from pyruvic acid. Thus
pyruvic acid was not directly used but was decarboxylated and reduced
through several steps.

The operation of the tricarboxylic acid cycle in brain was demonstrated
by Banga *et al.* (1959) who succeeded in showing that the addition of fumaric
acid or other C_4-dicarboxylic acid was needed for the oxidation of pyruvate
by a dialysed dispersion of pigeon or rabbit-brain. Krebs and Eggleston
(1940) showed later that minced sheep brain formed α-ketoglutarate and
citrate from oxaloacetate.

The individual enzymes participating in the tricarboxylic acid cycle are
localised in the mitochondrial inner membrane and matrix (Figure 3.19).

Starting from pyruvic acid, pyruvate dehydrogenase (decarboxylase), an enzyme complex catalyses the oxidative decarboxylation of pyruvate in the presence of NAD, CoA, thiamine pyrophosphate, lipoic acid and Mg^{2+}, yielding acetyl-CoA, carbon dioxide and NADH. Thiamine pyrophosphate, the coenzyme of decarboxylase and lipoate transfers hydrogen from the substrate to NAD. The latter reaction, which will be discussed in detail, when dealing with terminal oxidation, is catalysed by a flavoprotein called lipoamide dehydrogenase, which exists in multiple forms.

The enzyme synthesising citric acid from acetyl-CoA and oxaloacetate is called condensing enzyme. Among tissues assayed for condensing enzyme

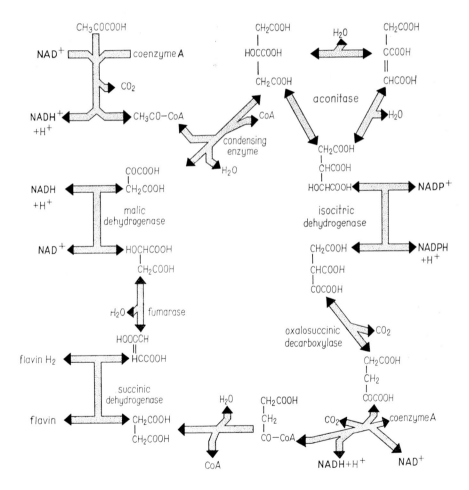

Figure 3.19. Tricarboxylic acid cycle

activity, cerebral tissue was found to be the most active (Ochoa 1954). Condensing enzyme activity was present in tumours in amounts comparable to the levels in normal tissue (Wenner et al. 1952).

The next step consists of the isomerisation of citric acid to isocitric acid through the intermediate of cis-aconitic acid. This reaction is catalysed by aconitase and inhibited by fluorocitrate. Aconitase activity was found by Wenner et al. (1952) to be lower in mouse hepatoma and adenocarcinoma than in normal mouse tissue. When fluoroacetate is added in vivo, the citrate concentration is raised in all normal tissues except liver and in tumours (Potter and Busch 1950). Aconitase activity was also inhibited in tumour tissue slices after the addition of fluoroacetate (Busch and Nair 1957).

Isocitrate dehydrogenase catalyses the oxidation of isocitrate to oxalo-succinate in the presence of Mn^{2+}. Isocitrate dehydrogenase occurs in two main types, that is, in NAD and NADP dependent forms. The NAD dependent form prevails in yeast whereas the NADP dependent predominates in animal tissues (Kornberg and Pricher 1951). Hence the latter enzyme was investigated far more in tumour tissue.

NADP dependent isocitrate dehydrogenase activity has been found in brain, but its activity was much lower than in kidney, liver and heart (Adler et al. 1939). The activity in the mitochondrial fraction was twice that in the supernatant. Some NAD linked activity was also demonstrated in brain by Vignais and Vignais (1961). In a comparison of the isocitrate dehydrogenase activity of ganglion and oligodendroglial cells, the activity of the latter was somewhat higher (Davison 1965). This may be related to the increased activity found in gliomas.

Rat tissue contains three or four isoenzymes of NADP dependent iso-citric acid dehydrogenase (Tsao 1960, Bell and Baron 1962). In brain only one isoenzyme could be detected, the same isoenzyme was present in human carcinoma. Although skeletal and heart muscle had different patterns, the demonstration of isocitric acid dehydrogenase isoenzymes in serum could not be applied for diagnostic purposes, because it disappeared very rapidly from the circulation (Standjord et al. 1960).

Perria et al. (1964) investigated both types of isocitric acid dehydrogenase in human brain tumours and normal frontal cortex by microchemical and histochemical methods. They found higher values compared with the normal brain cortex, measuring NADP linked isocitric acid dehydrogenase activity in medulloblastoma, spongioblastoma, astrocytoma and neurinoma. Oligo-dendroglioma, glioblastoma, ependymoma and meningioma showed activ-ities comparable to normal brain. NAD linked isocitric acid dehydrogenase was particularly high in medulloblastoma, glioblastoma and atypical astro-cytoma, followed by spongioblastoma and neurinoma. Oligodendroglioma, ependymoma and meningioma displayed activities similar to normal human cortex. NADP bound isocitric acid dehydrogenase activity was ten times greater than the NAD linked enzyme activity in the frontal brain cortex, but the increase of tumour enzyme activity was relatively higher in the NAD linked isocitric acid dehydrogenase activity compared with the NADP bound enzyme.

Lehrer (1962) found that isocitric acid dehydrogenase activity showed little variation in gliomas measured by microchemical methods, except in a well differentiated astrocytoma where it was relatively high.

Chason et al. (1963) observed a slight increase of NAD linked isocitric acid dehydrogenase activity in neoplastic tissue and reactive astrocytes. Rubinstein et al. (1962a) reported interesting data on the increased activity of NADH dependent isocitric acid dehydrogenase activity in the reactive macrophage system in cerebral tissue necrosis. NAD dependent isocitric acid dehydrogenase activity was shown to be reduced in experimentally induced ependymomas except in the tumour cells close to brain parenchyma (Rubinstein et al. 1965). In large anaplastic tumour cells of gliomas and metastatic brain carcinoma they observed an increase of NADP dependent isocitric acid dehydrogenase (Rubinstein and Sutton 1964). The increase of NADP linked isocitric acid dehydrogenase activity is important in fat metabolism, since isocitrate and NADPH have been shown to be necessary cofactors in fatty acid synthesis (Porter and Folch 1957).

The decarboxylation of oxalosuccinate to ketoglutarate proceeds spontaneously to some extent but is catalysed in brain by oxalosuccinate carboxylase (Ochoa 1948), whereas in other tissues this step and the dehydrogenation of isocitric acid could not be separated. The equilibrium of the decarboxylation is far on the side of the ketoglutarate formation, although starting from ketoglutarate, carbon dioxide and reduced NADP. Ochoa (1948) demonstrated the reversibility of the reaction in other tissues, thus the possibility of carbon dioxide fixation is given.

For the further metabolism of α-ketoglutarate there still exists two possibilities in the brain. Its relation to glutamic acid and the so-called GABA shunt will be discussed in the section on amino acid metabolism. In the Krebs cycle ketoglutarate undergoes a dismutation similar to that of pyruvate, which is catalysed by an enzyme complex called ketoglutarate dehydrogenase or oxidase. This enzyme requires in the first step NAD and CoA besides the substrate yielding succinyl-CoA, carbon dioxide and reduced NAD. Succinyl-CoA, like acetyl-CoA, contains a high energy acyl group bond which is transformed in the presence of GDP and inorganic phosphate to GTP, succinate and CoA. Thiamine pyrophosphate and lipoic acid possibly play the same rôle in ketoglutarate decarboxylation and hydrogen transfer, as in pyruvate oxidation (Kaufman et al. 1953, Sanadi et al. 1956). The enzyme was also isolated from brain and demonstrated to act reversibly (Wollemann and Feuer 1956, Wollemann 1959).

The activity of ketoglutarate dehydrogenase in brain tumours has not yet been investigated. Hepatomas showed lower activities compared with liver and brain tissue from rat (Wenner et al. 1952). Ganglion cells displayed somewhat higher activities than oligodendroglia (Davison 1965).

Succinate is oxidised in the next step to fumarate by succinate dehydrogenase. This reaction is inhibited competitively by malonate. Succinate dehydrogenase activity was extensively investigated in brain tissue by Quastel (1939). It was found largely in the mitochondrial fraction (Aldridge 1953, Aldridge and Johnson 1959, Abood et al. 1952) and identified as a flavoprotein (Giuditta and Singer 1959). Recently Hajós and Kerpel-Fronius (1969) showed differences in the succinate dehydrogenase activity of the neuronal mitochondria localised in the perikarya and axon terminals. The mitochondria of the axon terminals displayed no activity although cytochrome oxidase was distributed uniformly in both types of mitochondria. According to the cytochemical data of Davison (1965) succinic oxidase, that is dehydrogenase, was found to be twice as high in oligodendroglia compared with ganglion cells. Hydén and Pigón (1960) reported that the glial/nerve cell ratio for succinate dehydrogenase was seven and this ratio was reversed in the Deiter's nucleus after vestibular rotatory stimulation.

Succinate dehydrogenase activity in experimentally induced carcinoma and human neoplastic diseases is low, but in the same range as the least active normal tissue. Rat and mouse hepatomas display a succinate dehydrogenase activity that is one-fourth of that of normal liver (Schneider and Hogeboom 1950, 1951).

Reduced succinate dehydrogenase activity was also encountered by several authors in brain tumours. Friede (1959) first reported low succinate dehydrogenase activities from human biopsies of brain tumours (four gliomas, one medulloblastoma and one chorioid papilloma) using histochemical methods. Similarly, slight or no staining was found by Udvarhelyi et al. (1962) and O'Connor and Laws (1963) in all investigated brain tumour groups (gliomas, meningiomas and miscellaneous intracranial tumours). Nasu and Viale (1962) and Viale and Ibba (1964) were able also to show a decreased activity in all investigated brain tumours by histochemical and microchemical methods, with a major decrease in the atypical and undifferentiated neoplastic cells of gliomas; only hypertrophic astrocytes displayed relatively high activities.

Ogawa and Zimmermann (1959) working with experimentally induced ependymoma of C3H mice found that the succinate dehydrogenase activity in the ependymoma was much lower than in normal cerebrum. A relationship has also been shown between the number, distribution and localisation of mitochondria and succinate dehydrogenase activity.

Rubinstein et al. (1965), investigating the intermediary metabolism of various experimental tumours after intracerebral implantation, found diminished succinate dehydrogenase activities using histochemical methods.

In contrast to the data of these authors, several investigators give accounts of increased activities of succinate dehydrogenase in brain tumours, especially gliomas (Potanos et al. 1959, Mossakowski 1962, Schiffer and Vesco 1962, Chason et al. 1963). Potanos did not find any significant difference in activity between oligodendrocytes of normal and neoplastic tissues. Mossakowski (1962) demonstrated that succinate dehydrogenase activity was present in all glial tumours. The activity was enhanced with increasing anaplasia of the tumours. The succinate dehydrogenase activity of piloid astrocytoma was similar to normal astrocytes in white matter. Succinate dehydrogenase in gemistocytic astrocytoma, malignant glioma and glioblastoma multiforme was considerably higher than in normal glia. Reactive glia also showed greater activity than normal glia.

Schiffer and Vesco (1962) reported elevated activities by histochemical methods in gliomas, especially in hypertrophic astrocytes. A high activity was encountered not only in the cytoplasm but also in the processes of astrocytes. Gemistocytic astrocytoma displayed variable activities. Giant cells of glioblastoma and spongioblastoma also showed positive reactions in the whole cytoplasm. Chason *et al.* (1963) demonstrated a moderate increase of succinate dehydrogenase activity in neoplastic cells, reactive astrocytes and oligodendrocytes of gliomas. They explained the contradictory results of Friede (1959) and Potanos *et al.* (1959) with technical differences, as do Viale and Ibba (1964).

In our opinion, the results can also be explained by the variable presence of hypertrophic reactive astrocytes in glial tumours, which all possess, relatively high enzymic respiratory activities. The great variation in tumour cells of the gliomas is also a cause of contradictory data. Rubinstein and Smith (1962) observed a strong increase in succinate dehydrogenase activity following experimentally induced cortical injury in cat astrocytes of white matter only ninety-five days after the lesion, whereas the other increased dehydrogenase enzyme activities reached their maxima within fourteen days. The reaction was stronger in reactive microglial cells in oedematous white matter than in cortical lesions. Smith (1963) also found that succinate dehydrogenase activity was strongest in reactive astrocytes followed by gliomas and normal astrocytes. According to our experiments (Wollemann *et al.* 1969) succinate dehydrogenase activity was moderately increased in the mitochondrial fractions of some gliomas, compared with tissue surrounding the tumour and normal brain tissue (Table VII).

Several attempts have been made to determine succinate dehydrogenase activity in cell cultures of gliomas (Kreuzberg *et al.* 1966, Gluszcz and Giernat 1969, 1970). The great variability of succinate dehydrogenase activity in tissue cultures was also recognised by Kreuzberg *et al.* (1966) who regarded it as a sign of malignancy. Gluszcz and Giernat (1969, 1970) reported strong succinate dehydrogenase activity in polymorphous anaplastic gliomas with atypical giant cells. Monstrocellular malignant displastic gliomas showed intermediate enzymic activity and non-malignant displastic gliomas composed of giant cytoplasm rich cells, displayed low succinate dehydrogenase activity.

The next enzyme in the Krebs cycle, fumarase, converts fumaric acid to malic acid. Its turnover is relatively high in brain, where it is firmly bound to the mitochondrial fraction (Shepherd and Kalnitsky 1954). Fumarase activity was present in tumours (hepatoma and adenocarcinoma) in amounts comparable to the levels in normal liver and brain tissue (Wenner *et al.* 1952). Viale and Ibba (1964) reported a reduced fumarase activity in all investigated brain tumours compared with the normal frontal cortex. Lowest values were found in spongioblastoma and atypical glioma. Highest values were displayed by typical astrocytes.

Malate dehydrogenase was found to be very active in brain tissue by Green (1936). Two different enzymes are known under this name, the first is NAD dependent and transforms malate to oxaloacetate thus closing the Krebs cycle; the other, also named malic enzyme, is NADP linked and forms pyruvate from malic acid by simultaneous dehydrogenation and decarboxylation.

The NAD bound enzyme was identified in two different molecular forms; one form exists in mitochondria and the other in the cytoplasm of rat liver

TABLE VII

SDH activity* of mitochondrial fractions of brain tumours
(A) and tumour surrounding tissues (B)

	Δ OD/mg protein	
	A	B
Astrocytoma		
No. 33	1.57	1.97
No. 87	1.02	
No. 25	1.02	1.08
No. 106	0.81	
Oligodendroglioma		
No. 78	0.73	
No. 123	0.32	
Glioblastoma		
No. 79	0.81	
No. 258	0.4	0.9
Ependymoma		
No. 84	0.85	
No. 145	0.29	
Spongioblastoma		
No. 105	1.09	1.24
No. 38	1.01	0.64
Plexus papilloma		
No. 127	0.75	0.39
No. 249	0.62	
Meningioma	0.56	
Temporal lobe		
No. 104	0.9	
No. 211	0.65	

*SDH activity was measured according to Slater (1963).

and brain as described by Delbrück *et al.* (1959). The malate dehydrogenase in the cytopla·m differs kinetically from the mitcchcndrial enzyme in that it is more sensitive to substrate (malate) inhibition and less sensitive to product (oxaloacetate) inhibition (Kaplan 1963). From these inhibitions it is evident that the reduction of oxaloacetate is prevented in the mito-chondria and the oxidation of malate in the cytoplasm. This enables malate to enter the mitochondria from the cytoplasm and oxaloacetate to be released into the cytoplasm.

Johnson (1962) observed that 45% of the malate dehydrogenase activity of rat brain homogenates appeared in the soluble fraction, while 40% was associated with the mitochondria. The remaining particulate bound activity may be released on treatment with water and therefore is possibly a cyto-plasmic enzyme occluded in pieces of incompletely disintegrated particulate fractions.

The purified mitochondrial malate dehydrogenase consists of several electrophoretically distinct components, which occur in varying proportions in the different organs and species. The soluble enzyme exhibits only one active fraction (Grimm ard Doherty 1961, Thorne *et al.* 1963).

Contradictory results have been reported on the differences between the catalytic properties of the isoenzymes from rat liver and brain mitochondrial dehydrogenase. Whereas liver mitochondrial malate dehydrogenase was reported by Mann and Vestling (1968) to occur in a dimer form, Thorne and Dent (1970) showed in brain mitochondrial preparations the interconversion of the isoenzymes, with full retention of activity. The latter findings and analyses of peptide maps (Dévényi *et al.* 1966) led Kitto *et al.* (1970) to suggest that mitochondrial malate dehydrogenase is composed of two similar if not identical subunits and that the multiple electrophoretic forms did not differ in primary structure but resulted from conformational differences. They proposed the name 'conformers' for this multiple form.

Although Vessel and Bearn first observed in 1957 the heterogeneity of malate dehydrogenase in human serum and erythrocytes, further investigations in human tissues by Yakulis *et al.* (1962) showed in all cases except erythrocytes identical patterns with malate dehydrogenase concentrated in two bands. They were unable to detect any specific changes in the sera of patients with elevated serum malate dehydrogenase activities and concluded that determination of the isoenzyme pattern has little value in diagnosis. Kamaryt and Zazvorka (1964) showed a fourth anodal band from homogenates of human heart, liver and serum.

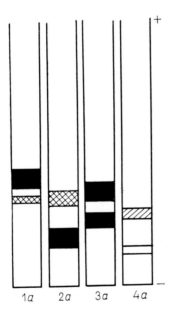

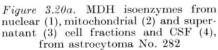

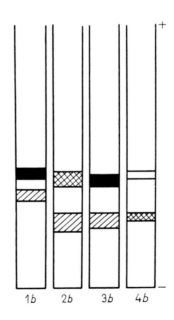

Figure 3.20a. MDH isoenzymes from nuclear (1), mitochondrial (2) and supernatant (3) cell fractions and CSF (4), from astrocytoma No. 282

Figure 3.20b. MDH isoenzymes from nuclear (1), mitochondrial (2) and supernatant (3) cell fractions and CSF (4) from medulloblastoma No. 279

Lowenthal *et al.* (1961) separated soluble malate dehydrogenase from human and sheep grey and white matter into six isoenzymes which were very similar to those found in the CSF. Van der Helm (1962) found no differences in isoenzyme patterns of malate dehydrogenase from different parts of human brain.

Comparing the malate dehydrogenase activity from experimentally induced hepatoma with normal liver, lower activities were only observed in homogenates with low NAD concentrations (Wenner *et al.* 1951). After the addition of NAD, normal activities were encountered.

Paxton (1959) measured NAD linked malate dehydrogenase by quantitative histochemical methods and found highest values in normal brain homogenates. Among the investigated brain tumours, glioblastoma had the highest activity and ependymcma, astrocytoma and meningioma displayed equally low activities. Chason *et al.* (1963) reported a slight increase in NAD linked malate dehydrogenase activity in neoplastic cells and reactive astrocytes.

According to Perria *et al.* (1964) NAD linked malate dehydrogenase activity was relatively high in the differentiated astrocytomas, glioblastoma and neurinoma. Ependymoma, oligodendroglioma and meningioma displayed lower activities compared with normal frontal cortex using microchemical methods. In atypical cells they demonstrated lower activities by histochemical methods than in differentiated tumour cells.

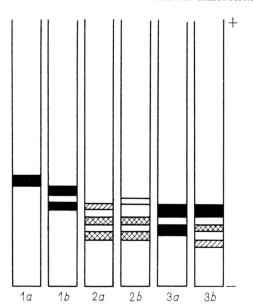

Figure 3.20c. MDH isoenzymes from tumour surrounding tissue (*a*) and tumour (*b*) of glioblastoma multiforme No. 258, nuclear (1), mitochondrial (2) and supernatant (3) cell fractions

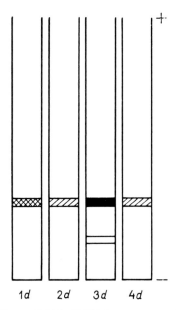

Figure 3.20d. MDH isoenzymes of tissue cultures of glioblastoma No. 258 (1) and meningioma endothel. No. 261 (2), cyst (3) and CSF (4) of oligodendroglioma No. 265

In our brain tumour material, NAD bound malate dehydrogenase activity was present in three bands in the heavy mitochondrial fraction of glioblastoma as demonstrated with disc gel electrophoresis (Figure 3.20c). Cathodal bands displayed stronger activity in the tumour mitochondrial enzyme compared with the mitochondrial malate dehydrogenase activity of tissue surrounding the tumour. In contrast, malate dehydrogenase activity in the supernatant was stronger in the bands migrating adjacent to the anode in the normal (tumour surrounding) supernatant than in the glioblastomal supernatant fraction (Figures 3.20a, b, d, Figure 1.2).

NADP linked malic enzyme is an alternative pathway for malate oxidation. The reaction product is pyruvate, dehydrogenation and decarboxylation occur simultaneously and are similar to pyruvate and ketoglutarate oxidation. The malic enzyme activity of brain is similar to that of heart, liver and kidney. According to Perria et al. (1964) malic enzyme activity in brain tumours is even more elevated than NAD linked malate dehydrogenase activity. Glioblastoma and astrocytoma displayed highest values. Malate dehydrogenase activity was also increased in various experimental tumours after intracerebral implantation as reported by Rubinstein et al. (1966). Cumings (1962) found no consistent changes in mitochondrial and soluble malic dehydrogenase activity of oedematous brain cell fractions.

3.5. TERMINAL OXIDATION

Enzymes responsible for terminal oxidation are also present in brain mitochondria. Mitochondrial fragments and electron transport particles produced by ultrasonic and detergent treatment of brain mitochondria showed oxidative phosphorylation and terminal oxidation respectively. (Abood and Alexander 1957). Electron microscopy has demonstrated that brain mitochondrial fractions centrifuged from homogenates (Brody and Bain 1952) are not as uniform as liver mitochondria fractions (Hogeboom and Schneider 1951). Therefore subfractionation by density gradient centrifugation (Whittaker 1959, De Robertis et al. 1962) and use of media other than sucrose is highly advisable.

Brain mitochondria display oxidative phosphorylation that is phosphorylation coupled to respiration. The ratio of esterified phosphorus to oxygen consumed (P/O) was comparable in brain mitochondria with the P/O ratio found in other tissue mitochondria (Brody and Bain 1952, Abood and Romanchek 1955). From the fifteen high energy phosphate bonds synthesised during the complete oxidation of one molecule of pyruvate fifteen molecules of ATP are synthesised. Among these, two molecules of ATP are synthesised at the substrate level that is, during pyruvate and ketoglutarate oxidation. The remaining high energy phosphate bonds (ATP) are synthesised during the electron transport, that is, reoxidation of three molecules of reduced NAD and one molecule of NADPH generated in the Krebs cycle by the flavoproteins and successive electron transport to the cytochromes. Succinate dehydrogenase being itself a flavoprotein reacts directly with the cytochromes and therefore gives rise to only two high energy phosphate bonds (Figure 3.21).

The NAD concentration of brain is one-half to one-third that of liver, kidney and heart (Glock and McLean 1955). About one-seventh of brain NAD is present in the mitochondrial fraction. The NAD content of brain is mainly in the oxidised form in contrast to NADP, which is over 50% in the reduced form, though the NADP concentration is low in relation to the NAD content (Jacobson and Kaplan 1957).

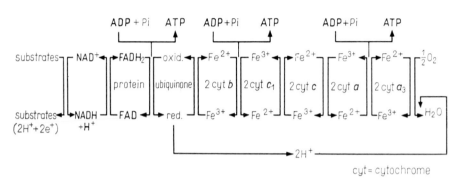

Figure 3.21. Terminal oxidation

Comparing the NAD and NADP content in normal and neoplastic tissues it is evident that the coenzyme concentration was in general lower than in most normal tissues. Glock and McLean (1955, 1957) found especially low reduced NAD and oxidised NADP levels in hepatoma, sarcoma and carcinoma of mice and rats. The NAD content of brain tumours was very low compared with normal brain and other tumours. Medulloblastoma displayed relatively higher values than glioblastoma. In the latter only the reduced NADP content was higher than in medulloblastoma according to Perria *et al.* (1964).

NADH cytochrome *c* reductase catalyses the oxidation of NADH by reducing cytochrome *c*. The enzyme is a flavoprotein and its activity in the brain is greatest in the mitochondrial fraction (Brody and Bain 1952). The other possibility of NADH oxidation is transhydrogenation to NADP, however, transhydrogenase activity is low in brain tissue (Kaplan *et al.* 1953).

NADH cytochrome *c* reductase was studied in homogenates of different tissues and tumours (sarcoma, carcinoma, hepatoma) by Rhian and Potter (1947) and Lenta and Riehl (1952). Enzyme levels in brain tumours were found by Perria *et al.* (1964) to be lowest in neurinomas and atypical tumour cells of glioblastoma, ependymoma and astrocytoma.

NADPH is reduced by NADPH cytochrome *c* reductase (Horecker 1950). It is also localised in mitochondria, and is called NADPH diaphorase, according to the original observation of Adler *et al.* (1939), who reported that dialysed extracts of acetone-dried tissue preparations catalysed the oxidation of both NADH and NADPH by methylene blue. Subsequently, a NADH and NADPH cytochrome b reductase was also demonstrated, but it was mainly localised in the microsomal fraction (Mahler et al. 1958). Succinate dehydrogenase may reduce cytochrome b directly; with the mediation of another respiratory coenzyme (ubiquinone or coenzyme Q) it may also reduce cytochrome c.

NADPH cytochrome c reductase was absent in hepatomas according to Reinafarje and Potter (1957). Perria et al. (1964) found similar localisation but somewhat lower activities for NADP diaphorase as for the NAD diaphorase in brain tumours. NAD and NADP diaphorases were slightly more active in meningiomas than in gliomas but the NADP diaphorase activity was particularly low in gliomas according to several research groups (Udvarhelyi et al. 1962, O'Connor and Laws 1963, Chason et al. 1963).

In contrast to these results Viale and Andreussi (1965) reported that NAD diaphorase and lactic dehydrogenase were the most active enzymes investigated by histochemical methods among oxidoreductases in brain tumours. Similar results were also obtained in cell cultures of tumours and in experimentally induced brain tumours (Osske et al. 1968, Schuberth and Kreuzberg 1967, Kreuzberg et al. 1966). One part of the enhanced activity is derived from the reactive glial cells. Originally normal astrocytes display low activities but reactive and gemistocytic astrocytes show high activities. The giant cells and small neoplastic cells also display a great variability in activity (Smith 1963). Rubinstein and Smith (1962) demonstrated a high NADP diaphorase activity together with other NADP dependent enzymes in the reactive macrophages of experimentally induced brain necrosis. As before, variable results can be explained by the different amounts of reactive cells.

The riboflavin of brain tissue largely occurs as flavin adenine dinucleotide in the different flavoenzymes, about one-fifth occurs as flavin adenine mononucleotide (Lowry 1952). According to Viale and Ibba (1964) the flavin content of brain tumours was parallel with their diaphorase activity, but among their published data (Perria et al. 1964) only glioblastoma showed reduced activity. Pollack et al. (1942), Robertson and Kahler (1942) and Shapiro et al. (1956) also reported diminished riboflavin contents in neoplastic tissues.

The presence of cytochromes a, b and c in cerebral cortex and subcortical nuclei has been demonstrated by their absorption bands (Huszák 1938). The cytochrome content of the white matter is low. Cytochrome c has the strongest absorption band and a low molecular weight (11 800). It contains a haem group bound to protein. The haem moiety contains protoporphyrin IX and Fe^{3+}. Fe^{3+} is reduced to Fe^{2+} by the diaphorases. It is interesting that the flavoenzymes also contain Fe^{3+}, which is reduced by the flavin-nucleotides and subsequently the resulting electrons are transferred to the Fe^{3+} of the cytochromes. The cytochromes are linked together in the brain tissue in the following order b, c_1, c, a (a_3). Of these, cytochrome b is also a metalloflavoenzyme and cytochrome a_3 is identical with cytochrome oxidase. They are inhibited by potassium cyanide and cobalt.

6

Among the cytochromes, cytochrome c and cytochrome oxidase are the most studied members of the terminal oxidation chain. The cytochrome oxidase activity in rat and sheep brain and other tissues was demonstrated to be present in excess of requiremenьs (Elliott and Greig 1938, Schneider and Potter 1943), but in human brain it may be a rate limiting factor (Hess and Pope 1960). Using microchemical methods the cytochrome oxidase activity was found to be mainly in the perykaryal region and in the dendrites (Hess and Pope 1960). Biochemical investigations using gradient centrifugation indicated a localisation at the inner membrane of the mitochondria (Ernster 1969). The cytochrome oxidase activity of white matter is considerably lower than grey matter (Hess and Pope 1960).

According to Schneider and Hogeboom (1951) cytochrome c is distributed equally between the mitochondria and the cell plasma, in contrast to cytochrome oxidase, which is localised entirely in the mitochondria. The cytochrome c content of rat brain mitochondrial fractions is only about 50 $\mu g/g$ compared to 90 $\mu g/g$ in liver (Klingenberg and Slencza 1959, Du Bois and Potter 1942) but the brain fractions are less homogeneous and probably contain smaller proportions of mitochondria. The respiratory activity of the cytochrome content of brain is the same as in kidney and liver (Drabkin 1950).

The cytochrome c level in neoplastic tissue is low compared to normal tissues with the exception of lung (Du Bois and Potter 1942, Schneider and Potter 1943). Greenstein et al. (1944) established that the addition of cytochrome c to an acetone powered preparation of neoplastic tissue pro uced more than a thousandfold increase in the cytochrome oxidase activity, whereas with normal tissue only a hundredfold increase was observed. However, decreased cytochrome c levels were not encountered by Chance and Hess (1959) in ascites tumour cells and hepatomas (Monier et al. 1959) as measured by microspectrophotometric determinations on the intact cell or whole mitochondria. Therefore changes previously described should be attributed to the loss of cytochromes during the preparative procedures. Cytochrome c was at least less firmly bound or metabolised more rapidly after tissue destruction in neoplastic tumour tissues investigated by Green stein et al. (1944).

In brain tumours cytochrome oxidase activity was also generally found to be low. Lowest values were encountered in astrocytomas and ependymomas; the highest cytochrome oxidase activity found in two oligodendrogliomas was about eight times that of astrocytomas. Using quantitative micromethods, the enzyme activities came close to that of the cerebral cortex (Allen 1957, Pope et al. 1957). This can be explained by the originally elevated cytochrome oxidase activity of oligodendroglial cells, which display 2–3 fold enhanced activity per unit volume compared to the Deiter's nerve cells in the lateral vestibular nucleus of rabbits and rats. However, after a vestibular rotatory stimulation this activity decreases in the glial cells from the original 3 : 1 glial neurone ratio to 1 : 2 (Hydén et al. 1958, 1965). Normal astrocytes display a lower respiratory activity. In contrast to these findings Viale and Ibba (1964) reported higher activities in astrocytoma, spongioblastoma, meningioma and sarcoma than in normal frontal cortex.

Lowest activities were encountered in glioblastoma and in neurinoma of the Antoni B type. Low cytochrome *c* oxidase activity was also demonstrlated by histochemical reactions in brain tumours by Udvarhelyi *et al.* (1962) and O'Connor and Laws (1963).

The histochemical reaction is based on the oxidation of *p*-phenylenə-diamine as substrate which is nonspecific, since ceruloplasmin (copper oxid-ase) and diamino oxidase (histaminase) also react with *p*-phenylenediamine. The application of the *p*-phenylenediamine reaction in gel electrophoresis helps to differentiate the three enzyme activities, since the different enzym-atically active protein fractions migrate various distances from the origin. According to our experiences with cell fractions of brain tumour homogenates the following changes are encountered after polyacrylamide gel electro-phoresis: two glioblastomas displayed copper oxidase, cytochrome oxidase and diamino oxidase activities. The first was localised in the supernatant and the others mainly in the mitochondrial fractions (Figure 3.22).

In view of the possible rôle of copper containing proteins in white matter respiration (Huszák 1947, Porter and Folch 1957), the high copper concentra-tion of brain tumours (Graschenkov and Hekht 1960) and the correlation of the copper concentra-tion with the malignancy of the brain tumours (Canelas *et al.* 1968) (see also page 42) it is also of interest to investigate copper oxidase in brain tu-mours. It is thought to play a rôle in some demyel-ination and hereditary diseases (Bennetts and Chapman 1937, Cumings 1959). Cytochrome oxid-ase also contains copper in the same propor-tions as iron (Yonetani 1960).

In summing up the differences of mitochon-drial enzymes revealed in normal and tumour mi-tochondria, they seem to be only quantitatively decreased. The cause of this change can be ex-plained by the decreased number of mitochondria per tumour cell (Allard *et al.* 1952). Wenner and Weinhouse (1953) also reported that the level of mitochondrial enzymes expressed in terms of nit-rogen concentration was lower in a miscellaneous group of tumours than in normal tissue. Similar data were also published by Hogeboom and

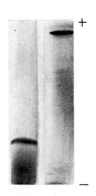

a   b

Figure 3.22. *p*-phenylene-diamine oxidase activity of glioblastoma No. 288. from mitochondrial (*a*) and supernatant (*b*) cell fractions

Schneider (1951). Electron microscopy of tumour mitochondria also re-veals altered mitochondria in brain tumours, for example, megamitochon-dria in oligodendroglioma (Luse 1962) and an altered mitochondrial struc-ture in cell fractions of tumours (Figures 3.23*a, b*). Loss of normal matrix and cristae, swellmg and bizarre configuration in mitochondria of exper-imental glioblastoma after chemotherapy were observed by Kirsch (1969). Tani *et al.* (1971) also described atypical cristae in mitochondria of human glioblastoma multiforme cells. Dohr (1961) and Dohr and Herranz (1964), investigating succinic dehydrogenase and cytochrome oxidase activ-ities of tumour homogenates and mitochondrial fractions, concluded that

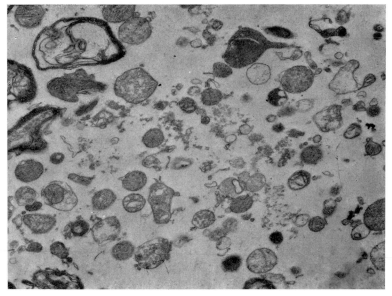

a

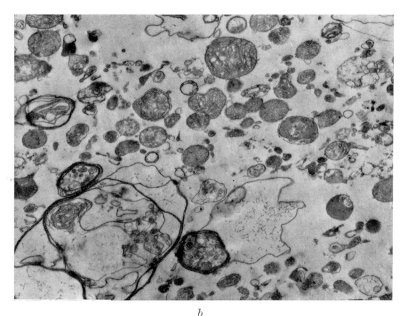

b

Figure 3.23a and *b*. Electronmicrographs of tumour surrounding mitochondrial (*a*) and tumour mitochondrial (*b*) fractions of glioblastoma
multiforme No. 258. Enlargement 18 000 diameters (Róna *et al*. 1972)

the decreased respiratory activity of tumours may be related not only to a decreased number of mitochondria, but also to disturbances in their enzyme system. The exact nature of these 'disturbances', however, is unknown.

3.6. METABOLIC REGULATION OF GLYCOLYSIS AND RESPIRATION

The first observations on the metabolic regulation of glycolysis came from Louis Pasteur (1876) in studies of yeast fermentation. He observed that in the presence of oxygen, yeast consumed sugar much more slowly than under anaerobic conditions. Since then, numerous studies have been conducted on different normal and tumour tissues and all of them displayed a more or less decreased glycolysis in the presence of oxygen. The phenomenon was called the *Pasteur effect*. The Pasteur effect in tumours is similar to that of normal tissue, if it is compared with the normal tissues having a relatively high anaerobic and aerobic glycolysis, such as retina, embryonic tissue and brain. In brain, the rate of glucose utilisation in the presence of oxygen is about one-third of that measured in the presence of nitrogen (Dixon 1937, Warburg *et al.* 1924, McIlwain 1959). Among the different tumours Ehrlich ascites cells displayed the highest Pasteur effect (Warburg 1956).

The reverse of the Pasteur effect was observed first by Crabtree (1929) and named after him. The *Crabtree effect* means that the addition of glucose inhibits oxygen uptake of tissues. It was originally observed on rat and mouse sarcoma. The inhibition is not large (10%) but increases to 50% using Ehrlich ascites cell tumour; some normal tissues, for example, renal medulla (20%), articular cartilage (54%) and postnatal retina (40%), also showed a Crabtree effect (Rosenthal *et al.* 1940, Cohen 1957).

The primary cause of these effects is explained differently by various authors. The first evidence indicated that the mechanism might be a competition between glycolysis and respiration for inorganic phosphate and/or compartmentalised adenine nucleotides (Lynen 1958, Chance and Hess 1959, Racker 1959), although the aerobic inhibition and rate limiting activity of phosphoglyceraldehyde dehydrogenase and hexokinase were also encountered (Engelhardt and Sakov 1943, Racker 1954, Wu and Racker 1959, Gatt and Racker 1959, Ács *et al.* 1954, 1955, Balázs 1963). The Pasteur effect is a very efficient regulation because energy production is about sixteen times higher during oxidation than during glycolysis. The reverse effect (Crabtree) is efficient only in the tissues where anaerobic and aerobic glycolysis are high and respiratory activity is low.

According to Warburg the main defect in tumours is the damaged tissue respiration. Indeed, one of the characteristics of tumour cells is the high glycolysis which coincides with a relatively low respiratory capacity. As discussed in the section on glycolysis, the isoenzyme pattern of the glycolytic enzymes is also changed in order to maintain a high anaerobic glycolytic rate. However, the primary alteration of these neoplastic changes should

Changes of Respiration in Brain Tumours

Enzyme activity	GL	GB	AC	OG	EM	SB	MB	NN	MG	MC	CP	EI
(A) HMP shunt												
Glucose-6-phosphate-dehydrogenase	+[6] +[1]		+[1]	+[1]		+[11] +[1]					+[1]	−[15]
6-phosphogluconate dehydrogenase			+[6]									
(B) Krebs cycle												
Isocitrate dehydrogenase	+[17] +[19] +[10] +[13]	−[11]	+[11] +[6] +[10]									−[12]
Succinate dehydrogenase			+[17] +[19] +[10] +[1]	+[17] +[19] +[10] +[1]	−[15] −[16] −[9] −[7] −[12]							
Fumarase			+[11]	+[11]		−[11]	−[11]					
Malate dehydrogenase	+[18] +[11]	+[11] +[18]	+[11] −[18]	+[11]	−[18]							+[16]
(C) Terminal oxidation												
Oxygen uptake	−[4-9]	−[2] −[3]	−[2] −[3] +[4-9]	+[2] +[3] +[4-9]	−[4-9]		+[2] +[3]					
Cytochrome oxidase	+[8] +[11]							−[8]	+[8] +[7]	−[4-9]		
NAD diaphorase	−[7] −[9]								+[9]			+[12] +[13] +[14]
NADP diaphorase	−[10]								+[10]			

+ = increase; − = decrease.

[1] Wollemann et al. (1969), [2] Victor and Wolf (1937), [3] Heller and Elliott (1955), [4] Allen (1957), [5] Pope et al. (1957), [6] Lehrer (1962), [7] Udvarhelyi et al. (1962), [8] Viale and Andreussi (1965), [9] O'Connor and Laws (1963), [10] Chason et al. (1963), [11] Perria et al. (1963), [12] Schuberth and Kreuzberg (1967), [13] Kreuzberg et al. (1966), [14] Rubinstein and Smith (1962), [15] Rubinstein et al. (1962a), [16] Rubinstein et al. (1966), [17] Potanos et al. (1959), [18] Paxton (1959), [19] De Risio and Cumings (1960).

be sought in the altered regulatory mechanism of protein and enzyme synthesis, that is, in nucleic acid changes. The respiratory alteration should be regarded as a consequence and not a primary cause of tumours.

3.7. LIPID METABOLISM

Most of the limited data available on the lipid metabolism of brain tumours have already been reported in the lipid section (see page 26), especially in the part concerned with the isotopic labelling of phospholipids and cholesterol synthesis. In order to avoid repetition it seems appropriate to deal here briefly with the synthetic and hydrolytic enzymes of brain lipid metabolism and with their changes in brain tumours.

The rate of turnover of the lipid constituents (cholesterol, fatty acids and phospholipids) of adult brain *in vivo* is very low compared to that of other organs. The uptake of lipids,however,is also restricted by the blood brain barrier (Strickland 1952). The small but significant synthesis of cholesterol from acetate-1-^{14}C and mevalonate-2-^{14}C in brain slices *in vitro* was observed by Grossi *et al.* (1958). Labelled cholesterol disappeared rapidly from other organs but it persisted for more than a year in brain (Davison *et al.* 1958, 1959). Klenk (1955) observed labelled fatty acids in brain slices using ^{14}C-acetate and Grossi *et al.* (1960) with butyrate-1-^{14}C, mevalonate-2-^{14}C and glucose-U-^{14}C.

Two main pathways of fatty acid synthesis have been hitherto described, one is the *de novo* synthesis from acetyl-CoA, via malonyl-CoA (Figure 3.24). In brain this pathway is confined, as in other organs, to the particle free supernatant fraction (Brady 1960). The primary fatty acid produced by this pathway is palmitic acid. The second pathway for fatty acid synthesis in brain proceeds through the stepwise addition of 2-carbon units to a long chain acyl-CoA ester (Figure 3.25). This system is localised in the particulate cell fractions. Aeberhard and Menkes (1968) found that acetyl-CoA and malonyl-CoA were the main substrates in the mitochondrial fraction, whereas in the microsomal fraction malonyl-CoA rather than acetyl-CoA was the active precursor in fatty acid biosynthesis. A significant amount of the fatty acids synthetised by microsomes and mitochondria was incorporated into phospholipids, triglycerides and cholesterol esters. The myelin fraction was almost completely inactive in fatty acid synthesis. *In vivo* studies on brain glycolipids also proved that long fatty acids are synthesised by a 2-carbon unit elongation of intermediate-length fatty acids (Hajra and Radin 1963).

Several fatty acids can be oxidised by cerebral tissue but only to a limited extent. Butyric acid and crotonic acids do not appreciably increase the oxidation of brain slices but octanoate-1-^{14}C and palmitate-1-^{14}C yielded labelled carbon dioxide (Volk *et al.* 1952).

The most active *in vivo* incorporation of ^{32}P was found in the phosphoinositide and phosphatidic acid fractions (Ansell and Dohmen 1957), followed by phosphatidylcholine, phosphatidylethanolamine and phosphatidylserine. The rapid labelling of the phosphoinositide and phosphatidic acids is supposed by several authors to be linked in an unknown way with membrane permeability and nerve excitation (Hokin and Hokin 1955, Larrabee *et al.* 1963, Hawthorne 1966). Due to the increased uptake of ^{32}P into the phospholipids in brain tumours (Selverstone and Moulton 1957), it is of great inteest to find which of the above enumerated phospholipid fractions is involved in the increased ^{32}P uptake.

According to Hokin and Hokin (1958, 1959) acetylcholine stimulates the uptake of ^{32}P into some phospholipid fractions. They therefore suggested that phosphatidic acids may be concerned in the transport of ions across the lipid membrane. The parallel increase of ^{40}K and ^{32}P uptake observed in brain tumours strengthens this view.

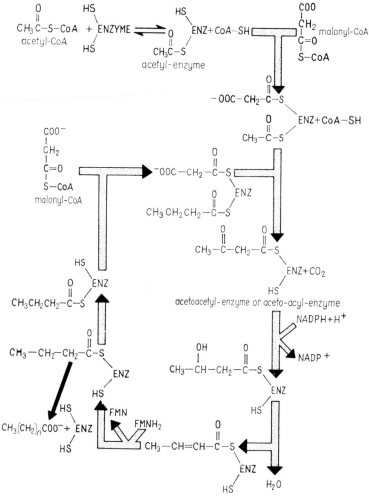

Figure 3.24. Fatty acid synthesis from acetyl-CoA and malonyl-CoA

The pathway of phospholipid synthesis in brain consists mainly of the esterification of glycerophosphate with two molecules of fatty acids to form phosphatidic acids (Kornberg and Pricher 1953a). Further experiments showed that cytidine triphosphate is necessary for the uptake of phosphorylcholine to phosphatidic acid thus forming lecithin. The intermediate compound formed from cytidine triphosphate and phosphorylcholine is cytidine-diphosphate choline (Kennedy and Weiss 1955, Strickland et $al.$ 1963).

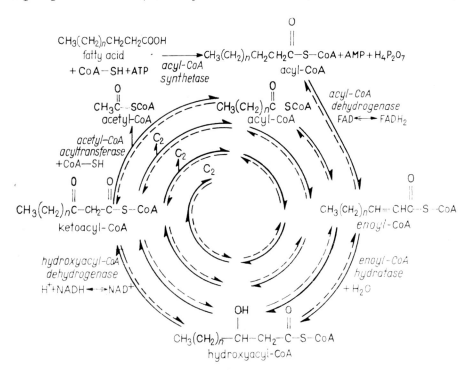

Figure 3.25. β-oxidation of fatty acids

There are few data on fatty acid oxidation in tumours. Both liver and hepatoma utilised octanoate in preference to acetate. Although normal liver converted more radioactivity from octanoate to β-hydroxybutyrate, glucose and glutamine, hepatoma converted more to glutamate, di- and tricarboxylic acids, aspartate and alanine. No C-2 fragments were converted to glucose in the tumours. β-oxidation of fatty acids to C-2 fragments and recombination of the C-2 units to acetoacetate or oxidation to carbon dioxide occurred in the same manner in hepatomas as in liver (Brown et $al.$ 1953, 1956). Hepp et $al.$ (1965) observed the aerobic formation of acetate in four different strains of ascites tumour cells and in one case of solid hepatocarcinoma, owing to decreased acetate thiokinase and normal acetyl-CoA deacylase activity. Weber and Lea (1965) reported that a decrease in biosynthesis and possibly a decrease in the breakdown of lipids occurs in hepatomas, correlated with the increase in growth rate.

With respect to lipid synthesis, authors dispute whether the activity of tumours is equal to or less than the lipid synthesis of normal tissues. It is certain, however, that the tumour utilises the fatty acids of the host (Henderson and Le Page 1959).

In brain tumours two enzymes of fat metabolism have been investigated in detail: β-hydroxybutyric dehydrogenase and α-glycerophosphate dehydrogenase. β-hydroxybutyric dehydrogenase forms acetoacetyl-CoA from β-hydroxybutyryl-CoA in the presence of NAD; α-glycerophosphate dehydrogenase reversibly catalyses the reaction between α-glycerophosphate and dihydroxyacetone phosphate in the presence of NAD and NADH respectively. The two enzymes are regarded as key enzymes of fat metabolism. β-hydroxybutyric dehydrogenase connects fat metabolism with Krebs cycle since acetoacetyl-CoA gives rise to two molecules of acetyl-CoA, in the presence of acetylthiolase and CoA. When the Krebs cycle does not function properly, or superfluous acetyl-CoA is present, acetylthiolase catalyses the reverse reaction and forms acetoacetyl-CoA from two molecules of acetyl-CoA, and one molecule of CoA is liberated. Acetoacetyl-CoA is in turn converted to β-hydroxybutyryl-CoA and used in fatty acid synthesis (Figure 3.24).

The synthesis of fatty acids proceeds mainly in the microsomes and cell plasma where NADH is more likely to be available, whereas in mitochondria the oxidation of fatty acids is dominant. According to Krebs and Veech (1969) β-hydroxybutyrate dehydrogenase is localised in the cristae of the inner membrane of the mitochondria, however, α-glycerophosphate dehydrogenase is present in the cytoplasm (Bücher and Klingenberg 1958). The mitochondrial oxidation of fatty acyl-CoA thio esters is strongly stimulated by carnitine-3-hydroxy-4-trimethylammonium butyrate which resembles acetylcholine in chemical structure. With the aid of two specific transferase enzymes palmityl carnitine is formed. Fatty acids are transported from the cytoplasm into mitochondria in this form because acyl-CoA does not penetrate the mitochondrial membranes (Fritz and Yue 1963). During starvation in the rat the β-hydroxybutyrate dehydrogenase activity of the brain mitochondria is increased ninefold. This indicates that when the carbohydrate reserves of the body are gradually lost, β-hydroxybutyrate becomes the principal oxidisable substrate in brain (Owen et al. 1967, Smith et al. 1969).

Lehrer (1962a), using microchemical methods, observed slight changes in hydroxybutyric dehydrogenase activity in gliomas, except for relatively high activities in two well differentiated astrocytomas. In agreement with Lehrer, Perria et al. (1964) also established that the β-hydroxybutyric dehydrogenase activity of tumours of neuroectodermal origin is similar to that in the more differentiated tumours and is absent in immature and atypical tumour cells. Therefore they concluded that the absence of β-hydroxybutyric dehydrogenase can be a sign of malignancy. On the other hand, Chason et al. (1963) using similar techniques to Perria, did not find any β-hydroxybutyrate dehydrogenase activity in any cells of the central nervous system, reactive astrocytes or neoplastic tumour cells.

α-glycerophosphate dehydrogenase connects carbohydrate metabolism with fatty acid synthesis. It occurs in multiple molecular forms in the mitochondria and in the soluble part of the cytoplasm (Bücher and Klingenberg 1958, Sacktor et al. 1959). Blunt and Wendell-Smith (1967) have shown that in the macroglia of adult cat optic nerve, there exists a glycerophosphate dehydrogenase which is not linked to NAD and is localised exclusively in astrocytes. This makes it probable that these cells play an active rôle in lipid metabolism, especially in the biosynthesis of phospholipids.

α-glycerophosphate dehydrogenase activity was found to be increased in reactive astrocytes produced either by local brain injuries (Rubinstein et al. 1962) or in experimental brain tumours (Rubinstein and Sutton 1964, Rubinstein et al. 1965). Smith (1963) investigated among other dehydrogenases α-glycerophosphate dehydrogenase activity in reactive and neoplastic astrocytes. She observed a decreasing order of enzyme activities as follows: reactive astrocytes, normal neurones, glioma cells and normal astrocytes.

α-glycerophosphate dehydrogenase activity is controlled by cortisol in adult brain and induced by corticosteroids in glial cell tissue cultures (De Vellis and Inglish 1968, 1969). Similar mechanisms probably take place during the formation of reactive astrocytes and their increased enzyme activities.

O'Connor and Laws (1963) reported variable activities in brain tumours. Perria et al. (1964) found a decreased activity in atypical tumour cells in agreement with Wattenberg (1959), Boxer and Chonk (1960) and Weber and Lea (1965) who found low levels in carcinomas, rapidly growing hepatomas and other tumours. Chason et al. (1963) observed weak activities in reactive cells and a mild increase in brain tumour cells. Gluszcz and Giernat (1969) reported that α-glycerophosphate dehydrogenase in short-term explant cultures of gliomas displayed activities similar to that of the original tumour. The degree of α-glycerophosphate dehydrogenase activity was intermediate between the NADP diaphorase and succinic dehydrogenase according to their observations.

The somewhat opposite effects of β-hydroxybutyric dehydrogenase and glycerophosphate dehydrogenase activities in brain tumours does not give a definite answer to the origin of decreased phospholipid content of brain tumours. Further investigations of other enzymes of phospholipid metabolism are needed.

Investigations on enzymes of cholesterol synthesis are also rare compared with the observations on the intermediate compounds of cholesterol synthesis (see page 28). The pathological changes in metabolite concentration are very often accompanied by enzymic alterations, but final conclusions cannot be drawn without enzyme activity measurements. The absence of a product, for example, might originate from a decreased synthesis as well as from an increased decomposition.

Besides the oxidation of fatty acids, special enzymes are known to catalyse the hydrolysis of the ester linkage in fatty acids and glycerol. Among these, lecithinase and lipase are not very active in the brain (King 1931, Webster et al. 1957). However in pathological conditions, such as demyelinating processes, their activity is enhanced (Morrison and Zamecnik 1950). Their possible rôle in the altered lipid metabolism of brain tumours has not hitherto been investigated.

Changes of Lipid Metabolism in Brain Tumours

Enzyme activity	Type of brain tumour	
	MT	AC
β-hydroxybutyrate dehydrogenase	$+^2$	$+^1$
α-glycerophosphate dehydrogenase	$+^2$	

+ = increased.
[1] Lehrer (1962), [2] Perria *et al.* (1964).

3.8. AMINO ACID AND PROTEIN METABOLISM

1. Glutamate and aspartate metabolism

The free amino acid composition of the brain is highly characteristic of this tissue and may be related to the nervous function. The concentration of free glutamic acid in brain is higher than in any other mammalian organ (0.01 M). Besides glutamic acid, other free amino acids occur in brain which are not present in significant concentrations in other mammalian tissues. These are α-aminobutyric acid, acetylaspartic acid and cystathionine; the latter occurs in the human brain and is the condensation product of serine and homocysteine (Tallan *et al.* 1954, 1958, Ansell and Richter 1954, Berl and Waelsch 1958). The pool of free amino acids is the source of amine and protein synthesis and also represents the products of protein breakdown. The dicarboxylic amino acids have the additional functions of partially compensating for the anionic deficit in tissue and binding ammonium ions by the formation of glutamine from glutamic acid.

The uptake of amino acids from blood through the blood brain barrier is very restricted in man. Glutamic acid, proline, lysine and leucine are not transported from the blood to the adult brain (Dingman and Sporn 1959, Lajtha 1958, 1961). In contrast, a net glutamine and tyrosine uptake from the blood was demonstrated (Schwerin *et al.* 1950, Chirigos *et al.* 1960). However, the exchange of free amino acids between blood and brain was found to be quite rapid, whether or not the blood amino acid concentration was elevated (Lajtha *et al.* 1957). According to the observations of Roberts and Tschikoff (1949) the free amino acid pattern in healthy tissue has a characteristic distribution when analysed by two-dimensional paper chromatography. In contrast, similar patterns of free amino acids were found in many different types of transplanted and spontaneous tumours. This reinforces the view of Greenstein based on different enzyme activity measurements, that the different tumours resemble each other chemically more than they resemble normal tissue, and more than normal tissues resemble each other (Greenstein 1954).

Investigations of the free amino acid composition of brain tumours by the paper-electrophoretic method failed to demonstrate the presence of

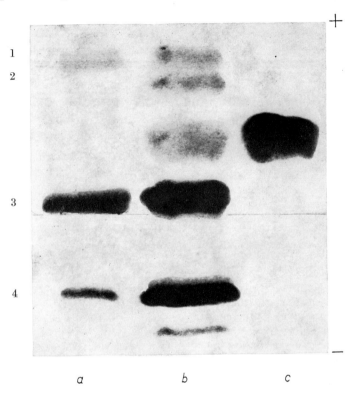

Figure 3.26. Paper electrophoresis of normal and tumorous brain tissue. Glioblastoma multiforme A. G. (*a*), parietal lobe D. A. (*b*) and GABA 20 μg (*c*); free organic bases (1), arginine, lysine (2), neutral amino acids (3), glutamic and aspartic acids (4) from Wollemann and Dévényi (1963)

γ-aminobutyric acid in any of the twenty-five brain tumours investigated (glioblastoma, astrocytoma, meningioma, neurinoma, ependymoma and metastatic carcinoma), whereas in control brain samples (frontal, temporal and parietal lobes, and cerebellum) γ-aminobutyric acid was demonstrated (Wollemann and Dévényi 1963). The sensitivity of the method was 5 μg. In the tumour material investigated, arginine, lysine, aspartic acid, glutamic acid and neutral amino acids were present (Figure 3.26) in quantities comparable to the normal brain samples. These data were confirmed by Promyslov (1969) who did not find any γ-aminobutyric acid or N-acetylaspartic acid in astrocytic brain tumours and concluded that these compounds are related to the activity of neurones and not to that of astroglia. However, Utley (1963) and Rose (1969) showed the presence of the GABA system in normal glial cells. Acetylaspartic acid normally occurs in high concentrations in the brain (80–120 µg/g) and is synthesised from aspartic acid and acetyl-CoA by an enzyme system in brain extracts (Goldstein 1959).

Lehrer (1962a) demonstrated that the glutamate content in brain tumours showed no marked differences from normal brain tissue but all values were lower than those obtained for cerebellar molecular or granular cortex.

Several enzymes concerned with the metabolism of free amino acids were investigated in brain and brain tumours. Starting from Krebs cycle α-keto-glutarate is transformed to glutamic acid by glutamic dehydrogenase. The equilibrium of the reaction in brain is in favour of the reductive amination of ketoglutarate (Strecker 1953). Glutamic acid dehydrogenase activity is localised in the mitochondrial fraction, mainly in the inner membrane and matrix (Sottocasa *et al.* 1967); however, 25% of the glutamic dehydrogenase activity is bound to the nuclear fraction (di Prisco 1970) in rat liver and differs in enzyme kinetics from the mitochondrial enzyme.

Glutamic dehydrogenase was crystallised from beef liver and was found to contain 2–4 atoms Zn per molecule (Adelstein and Vallee 1958). It was found by Frieden (1963) to exist in polymer and monomer forms. The active oligomer has a molecular weight close to 312 000. It is composed of six apparently identical subunits of molecular weight 52 000. The oligomer associates to form long linear polymers. Thus glutamic dehydrogenase is another example of an enzyme occurring in multiple forms. It resembles mitochondrial malate dehydrogenase (see page 94) in that the multiple form results from conformational differences. In accordance with this observation the electrophoretic data obtained by gel electrophoresis using agar gel (Van der Helm 1962) and starch gel (Markert and Moller 1959, Tsao 1960) are quite different owing to the different pore size of the gels. This transformation from polymer to monomer is influenced by various small molecules called effectors (Frieden 1959, Tomkins and Yielding 1961).

In order to understand the action of the effectors it is important to know that the oligomer catalyses the reversible oxidation–reduction of glutamate, whereas the monomer catalyses the oxidation–reduction of monocarboxylic amino acids, mainly alanine. Both NAD and NADP may function as coenzyme. ADP, NAD and NADP favour the formation of the oligomer, whereas ATP, GTP, NADH and steroids favour the dissociation. It has been demonstrated that glutamic dehydrogenase contains effector or ligand binding sites which are different from the active substrate or coenzyme binding sites. Therefore glutamic dehydrogenase is also classified among the allosteric enzymes (Monod *et al.* 1965). Glutamic dehydrogenase was one of the first enzymes in which a direct hormonal effect was found; namely, diethylstilboestrol caused disaggregation of the oligomer inhibiting glutamic dehydrogenase activity and promoting alanine dehydrogenase activity (Tomkins and Yielding 1961).

Carruthers (1950) recognised a greatly reduced glutamic dehydrogenase activity in cell fractions of Ehrlich ascites tumour compared with mouse liver fraction. Novikoff (1960) demonstrated by histochemical methods glutamic dehydrogenase activity in solid and ascites tumours.

Glutamic dehydrogenase activity was investigated in local brain injury and brain tumours by Rubinstein and Smith (1962), Rubinstein and Sutton (1964). After brain injury, in the area of brain oedema, an increase in glutamic dehydrogenase activity was observed in astrocytes within twelve hours after the lesion was produced. The NAD dependent form of glutamic dehydrogenase was found to be increased in reactive astrocytes, hypertrophic and gemistocytic astrocytes and giant cells, whereas no NADP dependent enzyme activity could be demonstrated. According to Perria et al. (1964) hypertrophic astrocytes and gemistocytes as well as gangliocytes showed the highest glutamic dehydrogenase activity, whereas astroblasts and atypical tumour cells as well as neurinomas displayed the lowest NAD dependent glutamic dehydrogenase activities. No glutamic dehydrogenase activity was present in proliferating blood vessels of malignant gliomas, metastatic carcinomas, meningiomas and medulloblastomas (Kreuzberg and Gullotta 1967). Oligodendroglioma, ependymoma and astrocytoma were particularly active. Brain tissue cultures of dysplastic gliomas also showed increased glutamic dehydrogenase activity with both NAD and NADP dependent enzymes.

Glutamic dehydrogenase was recently reported to occur in different forms in liver mitochondrial and nuclear fractions (di Prisco 1970). A different localisation of glutamic dehydrogenase activity in the various cell fractions of brain tumours and normal brain tissue was also encountered using disc gel electrophoresis (Róna et al. 1971) (Figure 3.26).

The next step in glutamate metabolism is its conversion to glutamine, binding another molecule of ammonia in the presence of ATP and Mg^{2+} (Krebs 1935, Speck 1949, Awapara and Seale 1952). The reaction is catalysed by glutamine synthetase and is very active in brain. The reaction proceeds in two steps: the first consists of the ATP and Mg^{2+} dependent binding of glutamate to the enzyme; the second is the reaction of the carboxyl-activated glutamate with either ammonia or hydroxylamine to yield glutamine or glutamylhydroxamic acid. The presence of ammonia stimulates the reaction and inhibition of synthesis has been observed after the administration of convulsant agents such as methionine sulphoximine (Tower 1960a). The glutamine synthetase is localised in the

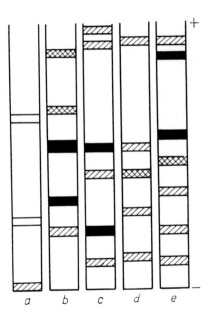

Figure 3.27. Multiple forms of GDH from crystalline beef liver enzyme (a), rat liver mitochondria (b), rat brain mitochondria (c), mitochondria of mesencephalon of twenty-eight week old human embryonic brain (d), glioblastoma multiforme No. 288 mitochondria (e). Activity stained according the method of van der Helm (1962)

microsomal fraction (Waelsch 1959) and in the endoplasmic reticulum (Sellinger and de Verster 1962).

Recently it has been shown by Holzer *et al.* (1970) that glutamine synthetase, like glycogen phosphorylase and glycogen synthetase exists in an active *a* form and an inactive *b* form in *E. coli*. The inactive form contains twelve molecules of ATP bound to the phenolic hydroxyl group of the tyrosine amino acid of the enzyme. The enzyme retains its activity after splitting the bound AMP through another deadenylating enzyme.

The reversible reaction forming glutamic acid and ammonia from glutamine is catalysed by another enzyme called glutaminase. Glutaminase is activated in the presence of phosphate or arsenate. In Ehrlich and Yoshida tumour cells relatively high levels of phosphate activated glutaminase have been found. In accordance with this observation, radioactive glutamine-2-^{14}C readily enters the tumour cells and is rapidly converted to glutamic acid (Roberts *et al.* 1956). Experiments on brain tumours are, however, still lacking. Brain glutaminase exists in three different molecular forms (Svenneby 1970).

Another possibility for glutamic acid deamination is its transamination to keto acids. Three transaminases act on glutamate and all use pyridoxal phosphate as coenzyme. The first is called glutamic-oxaloaceti transaminase (GOT, aspartate aminotransferase), the second glutamic-pyruvic transaminase (alanine aminotransferase) and the third γ-aminobutyric-α-ketoglutaric transaminase (GABA-T). In the first reaction glutamic acid is transaminated in the presence of oxaloacetic acid to α-ketoglutaric acid and aspartic acid. In the second glutamate is transaminated in the presence of pyruvate to alanine and ketoglutarate. In the third reaction γ-aminobutyric acid is transaminated in the presence of α-ketoglutarate to glutamate and succinic semialdehyde.

The two glutamic transaminases occur in most human and animal tissues. Since the transaminase concentration in the tissues is several thousand times greater than in blood, tissue damage leads to a marked enzyme activity increase in serum. This fact is extensively used in diagnosis; for example, myocardial infarctions lead to an increase in serum aspartate aminotransferase. While in hepatitis both aminotransferases are increased. Aspartate transaminase occurs in brain cell fractions in multiple molecular forms. One isoenzyme occurs in the mitochondrial fraction and another in the soluble fraction derived from synaptosomes (Fonnum 1968).

Alanyl aminotransferase is several times less active in brain than aspartate transaminase and its distribution is similar to the latter in brain cell fractions (van Kempen *et al.* 1965, Salganikoff and De Robertis 1965). According to Fleisher (1960) and Boyd (1962) it occurs almost exclusively in the supernatant of cell fractions of animal tissues and only one band appears after gel electrophoresis. This contradicts the findings of later investigations.

The determination of glutamic-oxaloacetic transaminase activities in the CSF in diseases of the CNS were not as conclusive as the results of the determinations in blood serum after heart and liver diseases. Green *et al.* (1957) found that the glutamic-oxaloacetic transaminase activity in the CSF was not significantly increased in any of the investigated primary brain tumours.

In later investigations the same authors (1958) reported elevated activities in ten out of twenty-four cases. Thompson *et al.* (1959) found the glutamic-oxaloacetic transaminase activity in CSF was within normal limits in brain tumours and other neurological diseases. No significant differences were encountered between normal brain tissue and brain tumour homogenates, which contradicts the data of Green *et al.* (1959) who found greater activities in the tumour homogenates on a fresh weight basis but much smaller differences based on soluble protein. Finally, Corridori *et al.* (1960) found that glutamic-oxaloacetic transaminase activity was increased only in a few cases of tumours and decreased in most cases. The increased activity was related, in their opinion, to the increased concentration of soluble proteins in neoplastic tissue homogenates extracted with phosphate buffer. Homogenisation in isotonic sucrose did not result in increased values for soluble protein in brain tumours (Wollemann *et al.* 1969). De Risio and Cumings (1960) reported no consistent elevation of glutamic-oxaloacetic dehydrogenase activity in brain white matter. These somewhat contradictory results could perhaps be solved by using gel electrophoresis and simultaneous staining of soluble protein fractions and isoenzyme staining. Otani and Morris (1965) found different isoenzyme patterns of glutamic-oxaloacetic transaminase in normal rat liver and hepatoma. Perria *et al.* (1964) found relatively high activities of glutamic oxaloacetic transaminase among brain tumours in typical ependymomas and low activities in glioblastomas. Unfortunately control brain values were not included.

The third transaminase involved in glutamate metabolism is γ-aminobutyric-α-ketoglutaric transaminase. It also contains bound pyridoxal phosphate as coenzyme, and it transaminates γ-aminobutyric acid in the presence of α-ketoglutarate to glutamic acid and succinic semialdehyde. Succinic semialdehyde is oxidised in the presence of NAD by succinic semialdehyde dehydrogenase to succinic acid, thus the so-called GABA-shunt from α-ketoglutarate to succinic acid is closed. GABA transaminase is localised in the mitochondrial fraction (Salganikoff and De Robertis 1965, van Kempen *et al.* 1965). According to Waksman and Faenza (1960) the GABA transaminase activity was decreased in one astrocytoma and two metastatic tumours and was similar to normal in one oligodendroglioma.

The enzyme involved in GABA synthesis is called glutamic decarboxylase. This enzyme forms GABA from glutamic acid by decarboxylation in the presence of pyridoxal phosphate, but it is less tightly bound to the decarboxylase than to the transaminase. Glutamic decarboxylase, like GABA is localised largely in the synaptosomal fraction and is inhibited by carbonyl trapping agents (semicarbazide, hydrazides, hydroxylamine) (Salganikoff and De Robertis 1965). Recently Haber *et al.* (1970a) used anions or aminooxyacetic acid as inhibitor to differentiate between the glutamic decarboxylase activity of cortical grey matter and that of glial cells, chick embryo, brain and other non-neural tissues. The neural glutamic decarboxylase was inhibited by anions and carbonyl trapping agents, however, the glial and non-neural glutamic decarboxylase was activated.

In an investigation of the glutamic decarboxylase activity of brain tumour homogenates (three glioblastomas, one astrocytoma, one meningioma and two metastatic carcinomas) and normal brain samples (two frontal, two temporal, one parietal and one cerebellar lobe), the activity of the tumours was between 0–10% of the control samples. After addition of pyridoxal phosphate to the homogenates the glutamic decarboxylase activity increased to 30–60% of the control samples, except in the metastatic tumours where the activity remained low (Table VIII) (Wollemann and

TABLE VIII

GAD activity of normal human brain tissue and brain tumours

Sample	Carbon dioxide production in $\mu l/10$ min	
	Without pyridoxal-phosphate	With pyridoxal-phosphate
Frontal lobe	52	55
	51	60
Temporal lobe	72	75
	65	70
Parietal lobe	41	55
Cerebellum	60	65
Glioblastoma multiforme	0	31
	0	26
	5	40
Astrocytoma fibrillare	3	32
Meningioma	7	15
Metastatic carcinoma	4	3
	2	3

Dévényi 1963). Haber *et al.* (1970) established that glutamic decarboxylase was lower in three cases of gliomas than in glial cells and white or grey matter, and belonged to the glial type, that is, it was activated by carbonyl trapping agents.

Asparagine was found to occur in a free form in nervous tissue in quantities well below that of glutamine (0.05–0.1 $\mu g/g$) (Krebs 1950, Mardashev and Mamaeva 1950, Tallan *et al.* 1954). Asparagine, like glutamine penetrates the blood brain barrier (Tower 1960). Asparagine synthesis in brain was demonstrated by Leshovaia (1954). Waelsch (1952) demonstrated glutamic and aspartic transferase activities in brain preparations using glutamine and asparagine respectively as substrates. Benuck *et al.* (1970) showed that the synthesis of asparagine from labelled aspartic acid proceeds in brain in the presence of ATP and glutamine.

Asparaginase activity in brain has been reported by Krebs (1950). In view of the recent results on the dependence of certain tumour cells for a supply of exogenous asparagine, asparaginase has been applied in general tumour therapy (Fidler 1971). No available data exist, however, on the asparagine metabolism of brain tumours.

GABA Metabolism

Substrate	Enzyme	Co-enzyme	Inhibitor	Product	Receptor	Inhibitor
1. glutamic acid	decarbo-xylase	PP	thiosemicar-bazide	GABA		strychnine metrazol picrotoxin
2. GABA + AKGA	transaminase	PP	hydroxyl-amine	glutamic acid + SSA		
3. SSA	dehydro-genase	NAD	diphenyl-hydantoine	succinate		
4. SSA	lactic acid or 4-OHB de-hydro-genase		K-oxamate	4-OHB		
5. glutamic acid	dehydrogen-ase + H_2O	NAD	GTP	$AKGA + NADH_2 + NH_4^+ + H^+$		

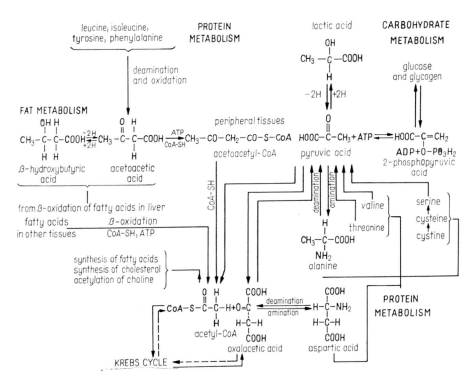

Figure 3.28. Relationship between amino acid and carbohydrate metabolism

7*

Glutamine and asparagine have been attributed with a rôle not only in ammonia binding but also in the increased binding of acetylcholine in hypoxia and in epileptogenic states of brain tissue (Tower 1960, Tower and Elliott 1953). Perhaps the decreased content of GABA and N-acetylaspartic acids in tumours also facilitates the appearance of seizures in some cases of brain tumours.

2. Metabolism of tyrosine and tryptophan

The metabolism of the two aromatic amino acids is very important in the nervous system since it gives rise to two highly interesting groups of neuro-transmitters, catecholamines (noradrenaline, adrenaline and dopamine) and indolealkylamines (serotonin, melatonin). Their function is central and peripheral, involving alertness and drowsiness, membrane hyperpolarisation and depolarisation, regulation of metabolism and contraction or dilatation of smooth muscles.

Catecholamines are produced in the brain from tyrosine by an enzyme called tyrosine hydroxylase which forms 3,4-dihydroxyphenylalanine (dopa). Tyrosine hydroxylase was first isolated and purified by Nagatsu et al. (1964) and shown to be pteridine, Fe^{2+} and oxygen dependent. The purified enzyme from beef adrenal medulla also converts phenylalanine to tyrosine. The enzyme is inhibited by tyrosine and phenylalanine derivatives (α-methyl-p-tyrosine, p-chlorphenylalanine), which are competitive with the substrate and with catecholamines, the latter being competitive with the pteridine cofactor (Udenfriend et al. 1965).

Tyrosine hydroxylase activity has been found in brain, adrenal medulla and sympathetically innervated tissues according to Nagatsu et al. (1964). It is particle bound, but Laduron and Belpaire (1968) claim that the enzyme is soluble and is adsorbed onto the particulate elements.

Tyrosine hydroxylase activity can be induced by different drugs such as amphetamine and reserpine (Mueller et al. 1969a, Mandell and Morgan 1970) and by exposure to cold (Thoenen 1970). In view of the fact that tyrosine hydroxylase is the rate limiting enzyme in catecholamine synthesis, its activity may be very important in catecholamine metabolism.

The next step in catecholamine metabolism is the decarboxylation of dopa to dopamine in the presence of dopadecarboxylase, first observed by Holtz et al. (1938) in kidney. The coenzyme of dopadecarboxylase is pyridoxal phosphate (Awapara et al. 1962). The substrate specificity of dopadecarboxylase is quite wide. Tyrosine and 5-hydroxytryptophan may also serve as substrates and their rate of decarboxylation remains relatively constant during purification from adrenal medulla, kidney and liver (Sourkes 1966). The enzyme activity is inhibited by α-methyl derivatives of dopa, tyrosine and 5-hydroxytryptophan, which inhibit the conversion of the carboxyl group to carbon dioxide (Moran et al. 1963 and Moran and Sourkes 1965), whereas carbazides and phenylhydrazines inhibit the coenzyme. α-methyl-dopa and α-methyltyrosine also act as substrates and can be transformed to α-methyldopamine and α-methyltyramine, respectively. These may act as false transmitters by binding to sympathetic receptors and stores, displacing the physiologically occurring catecholamines (Sourkes 1965). Owing to these actions α-methyldopa is now widely used as an antihypertensive drug.

Dopadecarboxylase is localised in the supernatant fraction from beef adrenal medulla (Hagen 1962), human phaeochromocytoma and human argentaffinoma. In the brain its activity is highest in the hypothalamus (Holtz and Westermann 1956).

Dopamine is oxidised further to noradrenaline in the presence of dopamine-β-hydroxylase. The enzyme was purified from adrenal gland by Levin and Kaufman (1961). It is a copper-containing protein and requires ascorbic acid and oxygen for activity (Friedman and Kaufman 1965). Ascorbate reduces the cupric copper of the enzyme to cuprous copper, which is reoxidised during the hydroxylation (Friedman and Kaufman 1965). The specificity of the enzyme is low and several other phenylethylamine and α-methylamine derivatives can be β-hydroxylated by the enzyme, such as tyramine, amphetamine, mescaline, α-methyldopamine and α-methyl-m-tyramine (Goldstein 1966).

Inhibitors of dopamine-β-hydroxylase are either structurally related to phenylethylamine substrates such as acetophenones, or are chelating agents, which act by binding copper (disulfiram, sodium diethyldiphenyl carbamate, α,α-dipyridyl, tropolones and phenanthroline).The *in vivo* inhibition results in high dopamine and low noradrenaline levels in the tissues and in the brain. The application of β-hydroxylase inhibitors in the therapy of neuroblastoma and pheochromocytoma is warranted according to Goldstein (1966).

Dopamine-β-hydroxylase, according to Potter and Axelrod (1963), is localised in the catecholamine storage particles. The enzyme is not freely liberated from the storage vesicles with catecholamines, but is localised between the membrane and the soluble contents (Viveros *et al.* 1969) in a sac-like structure (Belpaire and Laduron 1968). According to Viveros *et al.* (1969) reserpine, which acts by blocking the binding of catecholamines (Stjärne 1964), first causes a fall and then a rise above the norm in the dopamine-β-hydroxylase activity within 1–2 days. The enzyme activity increase is an inductive action since it is prevented by inhibitors of protein synthesis (Mueller *et al.* 1969, 1969a). According to Molinoff *et al.* (1970) the reserpine action is neurally mediated and blocked after surgical decentralisation.

The fourth important enzyme in catecholamine synthesis is phenylethanolamine N-methyltransferase (Axelrod 1962, 1966). This enzyme forms adrenaline from noradrenaline and it requires, like other methyltransferases, S-adenosylmethionine as methyl donor. The enzyme methylates normetanephrine, phenylethanolamine and hydroxyphenylethanolamine at a higher rate than noradrenaline. Besides phenylethanolamine methyltransferase, which occurs in highest concentrations in adrenal glands, there also exists a nonspecific N-methyltransferase in lung, which methylates phenylethanolamines and indoleamines. Phenylethanolamine N-methyltransferase is also capable of adding additional methyl groups to secondary amines like nor-

adrenaline, metanephrine and octopamine. Among them, N-methyladrena-
line occurs normally in the adrenal gland and in the brain. The enzyme is
localised in the soluble cell fraction and is inhibited by imipramine
(Tofranil®), a well-known antidepressant.

Apart from tyrosine hydroxylase and dopamine-β-hydroxylase there also
exists an alternate pathway of forming catechols from monophenols. The
catechol-forming enzyme was discovered by Axelrod (1963) in the liver
microsomal fraction of rabbit and requires reduced NADP for activity.
Tyramine, octopamine, sympathol and 5-hydroxytryptamine may act as
substrates and dopamine, noradrenaline and dihydroxytryptamine are
formed respectively.

The metabolism of the indolealkylamine serotonin is somewhat similar
to that of catecholamines. Serotonin plays an important rôle as a depressor
in the CNS and elicits the contraction of smooth muscle in the intestine,
stomach and uterus. Starting from tryptophan it is first hydroxylated to
5-hydroxytryptophan by the enzyme tryptophan-5-hydroxylase. The solubilised enzyme requires 5,6,7,8-tetrahydro-6,7-dimethylpyridine as cofactor.
Tryptophan-5-hydroxylase is localised in the synaptosomal fraction of crude
mitochondrial preparations (Grahame-Smith 1967).

The enzyme is inhibited by p-chlorphenylalanine, which causes a long
lasting depletion of serotonin and a short lasting depletion of noradrenaline
in vivo (Lovenberg *et al.* 1967, Miller *et al.* 1970). p-chlorphenylalanine
inhibits tyrosine and tryptophan hydroxylase, but tryptophan hydroxylase
inhibition is less reversible. Tryptophan hydroxylase occurs in high concentrations in the pineal gland in the brain stem, in carcinoid tumours and
in malignant mouse mast cell tumours (Grahame-Smith 1964, Lovenberg
et al. 1967). The inhibition of tryptophan-5-hydroxylase may be effective in
cases of carcinoid tumours, although side effects of p-chlorphenylalanine
treatment such as deprivation of sleep and restlessness in rats may also be
encountered (Koe and Weissman 1966, Jouvet 1969).

The next step in serotonin synthesis is the decarboxylation of 5-hydroxy-
tryptophan to 5-hydroxytryptamine (serotonin) with the aid of 5-hydroxy-
tryptophan decarboxylase. The enzyme occurs in all tissues where seroton
in is found, with the exception of blood platelets. The enzyme is highly substrate specific. Tryptophan, 7-hydroxytryptophan, tyrosine and phenylalanine cannot serve as substrate (Clark *et al.* 1954). It has a different pH
optimum (8.1) from that of dopa decarboxylase (6.9). The enzyme contains
tightly bound pyridoxal phosphate as prosthetic group and occurs in brain
alongside serotonin and tryptophan hydroxylase (Grahame-Smith 1967).
The enzyme activity is inhibited by hydrazines (N-(hydroxybenzyl)-N-
methylhydrazine) (Brodie *et al.* 1962) *in vitro*.

According to Arnaiz *et al.* (1964), 5-hydroxytryptophan decarboxylase is
localised within the cell, partially to the synaptosomal fraction, in contrast
to dopa decarboxylase (Laduron and Belpaire 1968) which is attached more
firmly to synaptosomes.

The serotonin content of normal human brain is highest in the pineal
gland, 22.8 μg/g (Giarman *et al.* 1960) followed by 2.0–6.5 μg/g in the caudate
nucleus, putamen, hypothalamus and limbic system. The serotonin content

of carcinoid tumours is high (Grahame-Smith 1964, Lovenberg et al. 1967). In contrast the serotonin concentration of gliomas and meningiomas is generally lower than adjacent cerebral cortical tissue (Joyce 1963). These results seem to be in contradiction with the eventual glial localisation of serotonin, although a contracting effect of serotonin on glial cells has been observed (Benitez et al. 1955, Geiger 1957).

The 5-hydroxytryptophan decarboxylase and serotonin deaminase activities have hitherto been studied only in hepatomas and were found to decrease as the tumour growth rate increased (Weber and Lea 1965).

The O-methylation of the catecholamines is the major metabolic pathway for the extracellular amines. Research on the enzymic O-methylation of catecholamines was stimulated when large amounts of an O-methylated product, 3-methoxy-4-hydroxymandelic acid (VMA), was excreted in subjects with phaeochromocytoma (Armstrong et al. 1957). In the same year Axelrod published an article on the O-methylation of adrenaline and other catechols in vitro and in vivo. He obtained a thirtyfold concentration of an enzyme from rat liver which formed metanephrine from adrenaline in the presence of the methyl donor S-adenosylmethionine, and Mg^{2+} (Axelrod et al. 1958). The enzyme was also purified from placenta (Gugler et al. 1970). All catechols such as noradrenaline, dopamine, 3,4-hydroxymandelic acid were O-methylated but none of the monophenols. This enzyme, catechol-O-methyltransferase, can be inhibited competitively by pyrogallol and other catechols and by the seven membered tropolones (Axelrod and Laroche 1959, Bacq et al. 1959). Adrenergic blocking agents also inhibit the extraneural catechol-O-methyltransferase in intact tissues (Axelrod 1966). These results suggest that catechol-O-methyltransferase is closely associated with the adrenergic receptor or has similar binding sites.

Catechol-O-methyltransferase is present in various tissues, for example, glands, blood vessels, sympathetic and parasympathetic nerves and ganglia, and all areas of the brain (Axelrod and Laroche 1959). The highest activity is present in the area postrema and the lowest in the cerebellar cortex. According to Axelrod et al. (1958) the enzyme is mainly localised in the soluble supernatant fraction but a small amount is also present in the microsomal fraction (Inscoe et al. 1965), which differs in some respects from the soluble catechol-O-methyltransferase. This enzyme should therefore be regarded as occurring in multiple forms (Axelrod et al. 1970). In vivo isotopically labelled experiments showed that about 20% of the circulating adrenaline was O-methylated and 25% deaminated (Axelrod and Lerner 1963). Almost all of the adrenaline or noradrenaline formed in the organism is excreted as the O-methylated deaminated product.

In subjects with phaeochromocytoma, there is an increased vanilmandelic acid excretion (Armstrong et al. 1957), and normetanephrine, metanephrine (La Brosse et al. 1961) and N-methylmetanephrine (Itoh et al. 1962) are also markedly elevated. Studnitz (1962) found an elevated excretion of homovanilic acid, vanilmandelic acid, methoxytyramine, methoxydopa, normetanephrine and metanephrine in subjects with neuroblastoma.

An O-methyltransferase other than catecholamine-O-methyltransferase is hydroxyindole-O-methyltransferase, which methylates indolamines at the

Catecholamine Metabolism

Substrate	Enzyme	Coenzyme	Inhibitor	Product	Receptor	Inhibitor
1. dopa	decarboxylase	PP	semicarbazide phenylhydrazine dihydroxycinnamoyl salicylic acid trihydroxycarboxychalcone α-methyldopa	dopamine	adenil-cyclase (β receptor)	
2. dopamine	β-oxidase Cu-protein	ascorbic acid	TM 10 bretylium	noradrenaline	adenyl-cyclase (β receptor)	ergotamine reserpine MMT propranolol
3. noradrenaline	N-methyltransferase	S-adenosyl methionine	methionine sulphoxide	adrenaline	adenyl-cyclase (β receptor)	tyramine dibenamine chlorpromazine
4. adrenaline	O-methyltransferase	S-adenosyl methionine	methionine sulphoxide pyrogallol quercetine	metanephrine nor-metanephrine		reserpine MMT tyramine DCI
5. adrenaline	monoamine oxidase		iproniazid phenylisopropyl-hydrazine nialamide isocarboxazide tranylcypromine	3,4-dihydroxy-mandelic aldehyde 3-methoxy-4-hydroxy-mandelic acid		only central: guanethidine tetrabenazine
6. 3,4-dihydroxy or 3-methoxy-4-hydroxy mandelic aldehyde	aldehyde oxidase	NAD		3-methoxy-4-hydroxy-mandelic acid		
7. adrenaline	polyphenol or catecholoxidase		adrenochrome			

Serotonin Metabolism

Substrate	Enzyme	Coenzyme	Inhibitor	Product	Receptor	Inhibitor
1. tryptophan	hydroxylase	reduced pteridine	p-chlorphenyl-alanine	5-hydroxy-tryptophan	adenyl cyclase	reserpine harmala alkaloids
2. 5-hydroxy-tryptophan	decarboxylase	PP	thiosemicarbazide phenylhydrazine α ethyldopa	5-hydroxy-tryptamine (serotonin)		mescaline bulbocapnine bufotenine yohimbine ergot alk.:
3. 5-hydroxy-tryptamine	monoamine oxidase		iproniazid α-methyltrypt-amine α-ethyltryptamine	5-hydroxyindole-acetaldehyde		LSD, BOL dimethyltrypt-amine, psylocybin
4. 5-hydroxy-indole-acetaldehyde	aldehydeoxidase	NAD		5-hydroxyindole acetic acid		

five position. The substrates of this enzyme are serotonin and N-acetylsero-tonin. The enzyme is localised mainly in the pineal gland and synthesises the hormone melatonin, which inhibits the oestrus cycle in the rat. Hydroxy-indole-O-methyltransferase activity is inhibited by exogenous light and by sympathetic nerve stimulation (Axelrod 1966, Brownstein and Heller 1968).

The intracellular decomposition of catechol and indole alkylamines occurs in the mitochondria. The enzyme involved in the oxidative deamination, monoamine oxidase (MAO), is located in the outer membrane of these orga-nelles (Sottocasa *et al.* 1967). Monoamine oxidase transforms monoamines to aldehydes. The enzyme activity is particularly rich in liver, kidney, intestine and the CNS. Metal ions and flavins have been suggested as co-factors of the enzyme (Sourkes 1958, Blaschko 1966, Gorkin 1966). Pyridoxal phosphate and cupric copper have been shown to be prosthetic groups of plasma monoamine oxidase (Yamada *et al.* 1963).

Investigation of the substrate specificity of the monoamine oxidase in various tissues showed differences between the applied substrates (adren-aline, noradrenaline, dopamine, tyramine, tryptamine and serotonin) for brain and liver. Phenylethylamines with α-methyl substituents acted only as competitive inhibitors (amphetamine, ephedrine, methamphetamine, α-methylnoradrenaline). Another group of inhibitors, the hydrazine deriv-atives, produce a long lasting irreversible inhibitory action. Examples in this group include iproniazid, phenelzine, phenyprazine, isocarboxazide and nialamide, some of which are used in the therapy of psychic depression. The harmala alkaloids produce a short lasting reversible inhibition of enzyme activity (Pletscher *et al.* 1959, Zeller 1959). Different inhibitory rates for the various substrates (catecholamines and indoleamines) have been encoun-tered, which suggested that monoamine oxidase is present in multiple forms (Gorkin 1966, Squires 1968, Kim and D'Orio 1968, Ragland 1968, Youdim *et al.* 1970). With the solubilisation of the enzyme it became possible to demonstrate the isoenzymes with the aid of gel electrophoresis. Up to five isoenzymes have been demonstrated in liver, brain and placenta, which differed in substrate specificity, inhibitor sensitivity and several other fac-tors. A different distribution of substrate specificity within the brain was observed. The dopamine oxidase activity of isoenzyme four of the hypotha-lamus was, for instance, several times higher than for other regions. In the uterus of rats the activity of isoenzyme three was stimulated after progester-one and oestradiol treatment (Collins and Southgate 1970).

The amine oxidase activity was investigated by Bülbring *et al.* (1953) in homogenates of eight glial tumours, one neurinoma and two meningiomas by the Warburg manometric technique. The activity ranges of the glial tumours fell within the ranges of the various parts of the normal brain, but the activity of the two meningiomas and neurinoma was well below these levels. The noradrenaline content was found to be particularly high in one astrocytoma from a three-year-old child. High levels of monoamine oxidase activity were found in pituitary tumours. Histochemical methods revealed small amounts of monoamine oxidase activity in gliomas, with the exception of the blood vessel wall, where high activities were encountered (O'Connor and Laws 1963). Kreuzberg and Gullotta (1967) did not find any activity in medulloblastoma. Unfortunately no data are available on the substrate used by Bülbring *et al.* (1953) for the amine oxidase activity measurements. Thus, in view of the contradictory results, no definite conclusion can be drawn about the monoamine oxidase activity in gliomas. Our own results on the monoamine oxidase isoenzymes of gliomas and foetal brain supports the view that monoamine oxidase activity is different in neurone and glial cells with regards to quantitative data and isoenzyme distributions (Figures 3.29*a*, *b*) (Wollemann *et al.* 1971).

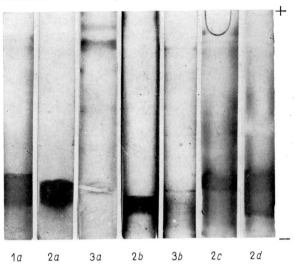

Figure 3.29a. MAO isoenzymes stained by the method of Glenner *et al.* (1959) using serotonin as substrate from rat brain (*a*), cat brain (*b*), glioblastoma multiforme tumour (*c*) and tumour surrounding tissue (*d*); nuclear (1), mitochondrial (2) and supernatant (3) cell fractions

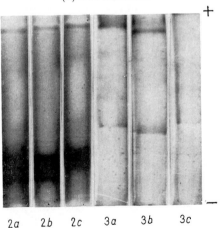

Figure 3.29b. MAO isoenzymes from twenty-eight weeks old human embryonic brain, mitochondrial (2) and supernatant fractions (3); cortical grey matter (*a*), mesencephalon (*b*) and thalamus (*c*)

The aldehydes formed from catecholamines (3,4-dihydroxymandelic aldehyde from noradrenaline, 3-methoxy-4-hydroxy-d-mandelic aldehyde or vanilmandelic aldehyde from adrenaline and 3-methoxy-4-hydroxyphenylacetaldehyde or homovanilic aldehyde from dopamine) and indolealkylamines (5-hydroxyindole-acetaldehyde from serotonin) are further oxidised by an aldehyde oxidase to the corresponding phenylacetic, mandelic or vanilic acid derivatives or to hydroxyindoleacetic acid. The aldehydes formed from catecholamines are not stable and therefore the specific enzymes converting them to the corresponding acids have been studied far less, with the exception of dopamine aldehyde oxidase which was reported to be a NAD-linked dehydrogenase (Fellman 1959). Weissbach *et al.* (1957) have succeeded in separating monoamine oxidase activity from aldehyde dehydrogenase activity. Besides dopamine-β-hydroxylase, disulfiram also inhibits aldehyde dehydrogenase, thus the enzyme probably also requires metallic iron for activity (Sjoerdsma 1966). Recently it has been shown that aldehyde dehydrogenase is absent from neuroblastoma (Goldstein *et al.* 1968), and therefore it was suggested that the aldehyde and alcohols formed in this tumour might be responsible for some of the toxic effects associated with tumours. In view of these investigations it is uncertain whether the different data on the monoamine oxidase activity of tumours are not a result of the lack of aldehyde dehydrogenase activity in the applied methods, which are based on the presence of both enzymes (monoamine oxidase and aldehyde dehydrogenase).

Stjärne *et al.* (1964), investigating the catecholamine storage granules from a surgically removed phaeochromocytoma, established that the tumour granules had a high noradrenaline content, while the adrenaline content was only a few per cent of the total catecholamine concentration. The ATP content was lower relative to the catecholamine concentration.

The pattern of urinary catecholamine metabolites in patients with phaeochromocytoma may vary considerably. Some patients excrete a low urinary 3-methoxy-4-hydroxymandelic acid / noradrenaline plus adrenaline VMA/NA+A ratio, exhibit a low adrenaline and noradrenaline concentration (less than 100 mg) and a small tumour, although the turnover rate of the catecholamines is high. Other patients exhibit large tumours and a high total content of noradrenaline and adrenaline (100 mg/10 g), a low rate of catecholamine turnover and a high VMA/NA+A ratio (Crout 1966).

According to Voute (1968) it is possible to differentiate between the different tumours of the sympathetic nervous system, neuroblastoma, ganglioneuroma and phaeochromocytoma on the basis of the excreted metabolised catecholamine products. An elevated concentration of homovanilic acid (3-methoxy-4-hydroxyphenylacetic acid) is characteristic of neuroblastoma and ganglioneuroma, whereas normal concentrations occur in phaeochromocytoma. He established that the patient who excretes only adrenaline, noradrenaline, vanilmandelic acid and 3-methoxy-4-hydroxyglycol has a benign tumour, patients excreting 3,4-dihydroxyphenylacetic acid, homovanilic acid and 3-methoxy-4-hydroxyphenylethanol, which are metabolites of dopamine, have a more malignant tumour, and those who also excrete metabolites of dopa (3-methoxy-4-hydroxyphenylalanine, vanilpyruvic acid and 3-methoxy-

4-hydroxyphenylacetic acid) have a malignant tumour, probably a neuroblastoma. The site of the block may be at different enzymes: dopa decarboxylase, dopamine-β-hydroxylase and phenylethanolamine N-methyltransferase may be blocked in different cases or an increase of activity of one of these enzymes including tyrosine hydroxylase is also possible.

Summarising the changes in tyrosine and tryptophan in catecholamine and serotonin metabolism in tumours of the nervous system, there are deviations in both directions according to the type of tumour cell: Tumours which are derived from nerve cells (neuroblastoma, ganglioneuroma) generally have an increased catecholamine metabolism, whereas the catecholamine and indolealkylamine metabolism of gliomas, meningiomas and neurinomas is generally decreased. To elucidate the site of the blocked or enhanced metabolism and the isolation and purification of the changed isoenzymes remains the purpose of further research.

Changes of Amino Acid and Amine Metabolism in Brain Tumours

Enzyme activity	Type of brain tumour									
	GL	GB	AC	OG	EM	MB	NN	MG	MC	NB
Glutamic-oxalacetic transaminase	$+$[4] $+$[2] $+$[9] $-$[3] $-$[1]									
Glutamate dehydrogenase			$+$[10]	$+$[10]	$+$[10]	$-$[6]	$-$[6]	$-$[10] $-$[6]		
Glutamate decarboxylase	$-$[8]	$-$[8]	$-$[8]	$-$[8]					$-$[11]	
GABA transaminase	$-$[11]									
Monoamino oxidase	$+$[5]					$-$[6]		$-$[5]		$+$[7]
Aldehyde oxidase										$-$[7]

$+$ = increase, $-$ = decrease.
[1] De Risio and Cumings (1960), [2] Fleischer *et al.* (1957), [3] Corridori *et al.* (1960), [4] Green *et al.* (1958), [5] Bülbring *et al.* (1953), [6] Kreuzberg and Gullotta (1967), [7] Goldstein *et al.* (1968), [8] Wollemann and Dévényi (1963), [9] Thompson *et al.* (1959), [10] Rubinstein and Sutton (1964), [11] Waksman and Faenza (1960).

3. Peptide and protein synthesis

The available data on brain and brain tumour peptide and protein synthesis are very scarce in comparison with some other organs and tumours. Owing to the blood brain barrier, the turnover rate of brain proteins could only be measured if amino acids were injected intrathecally (Gaitonde and Richter 1955, Lajtha *et al.* 1957). The incorporation of amino acids into the cortical grey matter was higher than in white matter, whereas with proteolipids, it was slow. Differences in the rate of protein synthesis between grey and white matter enable indirect conclusions to be drawn about the higher protein synthesis of neurones compared with glial cells. Similar results were obtained by Hydén (1962) using cytochemical methods on Deiter's nerve cells and glial cells. Among glial cells, oligodendrocytes showed a high incorporation of tritium-labelled glycine (Koenig 1958). Relatively large amounts of labelled amino acids were incorporated into the supraoptic and paraventricular nuclei of the hypothalamus, which play a rôle in neurosecretion (Richter *et al.* 1960). Investigation by differential centrifugation showed the incorporation of amino acids into the cell particles; most of the initial incorporation was found in the microsomes, whereas uptake by nuclei and mitochondria was relatively slow (Clouet and Richter 1959). Autoradiography with tritium-labelled amino acids showed incorporation into both the cytoplasmic Nissl substance and the nuclear chromatin (Carneiro and Leblond 1959). The protein showing the highest rate of incorporation was a liponucleoprotein in the Nissl granules, which are composed of ribosomal aggregates (Nievel and Cumings 1967). These data reveal that the active part of the microsomal fraction is the ribosomes. The incorporation of labelled amino acids into the ribosomes of guinea pig brain was similar if not higher than in liver ribosomes (Ács *et al.* 1961).

Inhibiting protein synthesis in brain by puromycin and cycloheximide produced memory loss in mice and fish (Barondes and Cohen 1966, 1967) and depressed electrical activity in isolated ganglia. Thus proteins are certainly necessary for such specific brain functions as memory. Puromycin binds the carboxyl terminals of peptide chains by forming peptidylpuromycin, whereas cycloheximide inhibits the growth and release of polypeptide chains. Chloramphenicol inhibits only the insoluble protein synthesis of brain mitochondria, while cycloheximide inhibits both soluble and structurally bound protein synthesis (Haldar 1970). As puromycin is the most effective memory inhibitor among the inhibitors of protein synthesis it was suggested that it blocks the expression of engrams by forming a peptidyl-puromycin-engram complex (Mayor 1969). Roberts *et al.* (1970) suggest that the peptidyl-puromycin is adsorbed onto adrenergic sites in the CNS and that these sites may be involved in memory trace. Protein synthesis is accelerated in sympathetic nerve cells by the nerve growth factor isolated from mouse submaxillary glands (Levi-Montalcini 1965). The nerve growth factor was purified and identified as a protein having a molecular weight of 29 000. It increased the biosynthesis of lipids, proteins and RNA in the sympathetic nerve cells of newborn mice. By producing an antiserum to the nerve growth factor it was possible to perform immunosympathectomy with the antiserum, which resulted in a 95–98% destruction of the sympathetic nerve cells.

According to Weber and Lea (1965) the protein metabolism of hepatomas increases with malignancy in favour of protein synthesis, thus an increase in the incorporation of amino acids correlates with the growth rate of hepatoma slices. The free amino acid level and amino acid catabolysing enzymes in hepatomas are not influenced by regulatory factors which may be hormonal (corticosteroid), nutritional (protein or tryptophan feeding) and by substrate induction, which are able to produce profound adaptations in normal liver.

Unfortunately little is known of the protein synthesis of brain tumours. Recently Seeds *et al.* (1970) investigated synthesis in cloned cell lines of neuroblastoma (*in vitro* culture of a single parent cell). They found that these cells have many of the properties of differentiated sympathetic neurones. The cells produce branched axons and bioelectrically active membranes which are electrically excitable and respond to chemical stimulation. Neurite extension was not inhibited by cycloheximide, but was sensitive to the addition of serum, colchicine and vinblastine. Therefore it was concluded that neurite formation depends on the assembly of microtubules or neurofilaments from preformed protein subunits (Seeds *et al.* 1970, Augusti-Tocco and Sato 1969, Nelson *et al.* 1969, Schubert *et al.* 1970). Protein synthesis in gliomas has not up to now been investigated.

A schematic survey of protein synthesis is given in the section on the metabolism of nucleic acids (see page 118).

4. Decomposition of peptides and proteins

Enzymic peptide and protein breakdown in brain has been known to occur for a long time. Proteinase with a pH optimum at 7.4 was more active in white than in grey matter, whereas acid proteinase (cathepsin) with a pH optimum at 3.8 was more active in grey matter (Ansell and Richter 1954). Investigating the subcellular distribution and properties of neutral and acid proteinases, Marks and Lajtha (1963) found that the highest activity of acid and neutral proteinases was localised in the mitochondrial fraction. On sucrose gradient centrifugation the neutral proteinases were associated with cell fractions containing myelin, nerve-ending structures and vesicles. The acid proteinase is presumably localised in the lysosomes. In a comparison of the proteinase activity of different tissue homogenates, the activity in brain was less than in kidney, spleen or liver but greater than in muscle (Marks and Lajtha 1963). According to Pope *et al.* (1957) the proteolytic activity in glial cells is of the same order as that in neurones. Weber and Lea (1965) reported a decreased activity of protein catabolism accompanying an increased growth rate in hepatomas.

Only four enzymes of protein catabolism have been studied in brain tumours: alanylglycine dipeptidase, leucyldehydropeptidase, leucylaminopeptidase and acid proteinase. The activities of alanylglycine dipeptidase and leucyldehydropeptidase in brain tumours were studied by Pope *et al.* (1957) and Allen (1962) who found them to be very similar. The activities of well differentiated astrocytomas and oligodendrogliomas were slightly higher than that of normal cortex and white matter. Ependymoma and medulloblastoma displayed low activities. Leucyl-β-naphthylamidase was investigated in native and cultivated brain tumour tissue by histochemical methods. In histological slides highest activities were encountered in neurinomas and lowest in glioblastomas (Matakas 1969). Gluszcz (1963) also observed high activities in medulloblastomas. After preparing cell cultures the activity in all tumours increased with increased lysosomal activity. Green and Perry (1963) measured leucine aminopeptidase activity in the

CSF of patients with brain tumours. They reported increased levels of enzyme activity, but this also occurred in a variety of neurological lesions and seemed to be no more specific than the frequently associated increase in CSF proteins. A high acid proteinase activity was found in two meningiomas by Lajtha and Marks (1969).

Burstone (1956) investigated aminopeptidase activities in human neoplasms with histochemical methods. Using 1-leucyl-β-naphthylamide as substrate, intense reactivity of connective tissue stroma, including ground substance adjacent to invasive epidermoid carcinomas, was found. In fibroblasts, polymorphonuclear leukocytes and macrophages, the zones of high peptidase activity were adjacent to the tumour) and not necessarily associated with an inflammatory response. Hess and Pope (1960) also observed highest hydrolytic activities in transplanted rodent tumours associated with macrophages, mast cells and fibroblasts. These data reflect a certain similarity to brain tumour activities.

Glenner et al. (1959) studying one hundred and twenty surgically removed tumours found alanylaminopeptidase in tumour cells from adenocarcinoma of the colon and stomach, melanoma and meningioma. Holmberg (1961) observed an in vitro release of cytoplasmic enzymes from ascites tumour cells. Thus protein catabolism of neoplasms is not a simple problem and cannot be investigated separately from the reaction of the surrounding tissue. Tumour cells and macrophages are probably involved together in the increased enzyme activities, and in addition to phagocytic reactions invasive tendencies are also present.

Changes of Protein Metabolism in Brain Tumours

Enzyme activity	Type of brain tumour						
	GB	AC	OG	EM	MB	NN	MG
Alanylglycine dipeptidase		+[1]	+[1]	−[1]	−[1]		
Leucyldehydropeptidase		+[3]	+[3]	−[3]	−[3]		
1-Leucyl-β-naphthylamidase	−[2]				+[5]	+[2]	
Acid proteinase							+[4]

+ = increased; − = decreased.
[1] Pope et al. (1957), [2] Matakas (1969), [3] Allen (1962), [4] Lajtha and Marks (1969), [5] Gluszcz (1963).

3.9. NUCLEOTIDE AND NUCLEIC ACID METABOLISM

1. Purine nucleotides

Adenine nucleotides have a multiple rôle in brain function. Adenosine triphosphate (ATP) may provide energy for various synthetic reactions, for example, amino acid activation for protein synthesis, acetyl-CoA for glucose and fatty acid synthesis, coenzyme synthesis, glucose phosphate synthesis, thiamine pyrophosphate, S-adenosylmethionine and cyclic AMP synthesis and catecholamine binding. The high energy stored in the phosphate groups of ATP can be also transphosphorylated to creatine forming creatine phosphate, which coupled to ATP, functions as another high energy store in brain. The reversible reaction is catalysed by creatine phosphotransferase (creatine kinase) which occurs in a multiple form. The enzyme is most abundant in muscle and brain and has a molecular weight of 81 000. Creatine phosphokinase was prepared in crystalline form brain by Jacobs et al. (1968). The enzyme consists of two subunits, which are designated MM in muscle and BB in brain and nervous tissue. Their amino acid composition is somewhat different.

Most likely, two genes are responsible for the synthesis of the two subunits, which may also form the hybrid MB. During ontogenesis the MM type in muscle changes to BB, but the BB type in brain does not change (Eppenberger et al. 1970). The BB type isoenzyme is also present in the CSF but not in serum (Shervin et al. 1968).

According to Shapira et al. (1968) the cancerous pattern of isoenzymes seems to be dependent on ontogenetic evolution and not on the type of glycolysis as reported previously by Kaplan (1963). Our experiments on creatine phosphotransferase isoenzymes of brain tumours did not confirm Shapira's theory, which was based on observations of LDH isoenzyme changes in hepatomas, where the H type appeared, as in embryonic liver, in contrast to the adult liver where the M type is present. Shapira et al. (1968) concluded that cancerous isoenzymic mod-

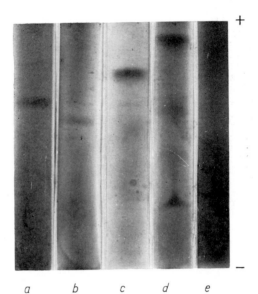

Figure 3.30. Creatine phosphotransferase isoenzymes demonstrated according to Deul and Van Breeman (1964) from normal human cortical grey matter brain supernatant cell fraction (*a*), embryonic human cortical grey matter twenty-eight weeks old (*b*), astrocytoma No. 318 cyst (*c*) and tumour (*d*) and glioblastoma multiforme No. 288 (*e*)

ifications reflect tissue dedifferentiation rather than a shift to an anaerobic glycolytic metabolism. The fact that creatine phosphotransferase remains unchanged in foetal brain and changes from BB to MM in malignant brain tumours (Figure 3.30) indicates that there are important differences between the isoenzyme distribution in foetal and neoplastic tissue, which points to an independent regulation of tumour enzymes induced perhaps by a virus-like ribonucleic acid dependent DNA polymerase (see page 117) (Wollemann et al. 1972). Most of the creatine phosphotransferase is localised in the cell plasma, but the mitochondria of liver and brain also contain some enzymic activity. The mitochondrial enzyme always exists as a single component (Jacobs et al. 1964).

Myokinase (adenylate kinase) transforms two molecules of adenosine diphosphate into adenylic acid and adenosinetriphosphate. It was discovered in muscle by Kalckar (1943) and later in brain. Similar reactions involving other nucleoside phosphates were observed later (Krebs and Hems 1953). Myokinase is known to exist in multiple forms in human erythrocytes, heart and muscle (Fildes and Harris 1966).

Lehrer (1962a) measured the creatine kinase and myokinase activities in brain tumours and found no differences from the normal levels. The breakdown of ATP in the brain proceeds mainly through adenosinetriphosphatase (ATPase) (see page 79 for the synthesis of ATP in normal brain tissue and brain tumours).

Brain adenosinetriphosphatase is localised in neurone and glial cells in two particulate cell fractions: mitochondria and microsomes. The mitochondrial enzyme is activated by Mg^{2+} and dinitrophenol. According to Tanaka et al. (1962) the Mg^{2+} activation was inhibited by fluoride and ethylenediamine tetraacetate. The microsomal adenosinetriphosphatase was described in crab nerves by Skou (1957) and in rat brain microsomes by Järnefelt (1961) as a Na^+/K^+-stimulated Mg^{2+}-dependent enzyme. The microsomal nerve cell fractions contained both nerve membranes and smooth reticuloendothelial fragments. The authors suggested that the adenosinetriphosphatase was involved in the active transport of Na^+ and K^+ across the cell membrane. The enzyme activity and the membrane permeability towards these ions is inhibited by similar concentrations of ouabain. Adenosinetriphosphatase is localised in the cell membrane with sites on both surfaces. Na^+ has a high affinity for the inside and K^+ for the outside and both ions are extruded: Na^+ to the outside, K^+ to the inside. Na^+ stimulates the formation of the phosphorylated enzyme intermediate, while K^+ accelerates the dephosphorylation. Ouabain reacts primarily with the phosphorylated form of the enzyme (Sen and Tobin 1969).

Cummins and Hydén (1962) found higher adenosinetriphosphatase activities in glial cells compared with neurones of the vestibular nucleus. The ATP content, however, was higher in the neurones. The Ca^{2+}-activated adenosinetriphosphatase in brain is of mesodermal origin and is mainly localised in the vascular smooth muscles, as is myosin adenosinetriphosphatase activity. ATPase activity was moderate in astrocytomas and meningiomas and lower in spongioblastomas, oligodendrogliomas, glioblastomas and neurinomas. The activity was not changed in tissue culture prepared from the brain tumours (Matakas 1969).

According to Hess et al. (1969) the presence of Na^+/K^+ activated adenosinetriphosphatase in astrocytomas suggests that astrocytes may have monovalent cation transport capacity. The results of Friede (1964), obtained on the enzymic response of astrocytes to various ions using tissue culture of rat cerebral cortex also confirm this view. Friede concluded that astrocytes are involved in the active transport of sodium, and he denied that astrocytes are formed from the oligodendroglia (Koenig and Barron 1963).

The distribution of ATPase in cell fractions of brain tumours has not been investigated. In hepatomas of mice and rats the mitochondrial adenosinetriphosphatase was decreased and the microsomal adenosinetriphosphatase increased in comparison with normal liver (Schneider and Hogeboom 1950).

Adenylcyclase, the enzyme forming $3'5'$-cyclic adenylic acid from ATP in a reaction which requires Mg^{2+} (Sutherland and Rall 1962) was originally discovered as an activator of phosphorylase in liver. The enzyme has been located in particulate fractions of rat brain cortex (nerve endings and synaptic membranes) (De Robertis et al. 1967). The enzyme is activated by catecholamines acting on the β-receptor, and is activated and inhibited by low and high Ca^{2+} concentrations respectively (Bradham et al. 1970, Straub 1969, Burkard and Gey 1969). Cyclic AMP is now regarded as an intracellular secondary messenger mediating many actions of different hormones. Besides catecholamines, glucagon, corticosterones, serotonin, insulin and luteinising hormones are also involved in altering the intracellular level of cyclic AMP; and a wide variety of enzymic processes, including lipolysis, protein and nucleic acid synthesis and phosphorylation, is also influenced (Robinson et al. 1968, Greengard 1971). Cyclic AMP also has several important functions in the nervous system. Melatonin production from serotonin is enhanced by the addition of dibutyryl cyclic AMP (Klein et al. 1970). Depolarising agents such as K^+, ouabain and veratridin enhance the formation of cyclic AMP from ATP (Shimizu et al. 1970). Reacently several papers have appeared dealing with the adenylcyclase activity of cultured human astrocytomas, meningiomas and gliomas which responded to all biogenic amines like normal brain tissue as well as virus-transformed astrocytes (Clark and Perkins 1971, Shimizu et al. 1971, Weiss et al. 1971). Dibutyryl cyclic AMP was reported to induce axon formation in mouse neuroblastoma (Prasad and Hsie 1971, Furmanski et al. 1971).

Nucleotidases are enzymes which hydrolyse both pyrimidine and purine nucleotides. Among them 5'-nucleotidase was investigated in brain tumours by Feigen and Wolf (1959) using adenylic acid (5'-AMP) as substrate. They found increased activity in ependymoma and astrocytoma. Normally it occurs in more elevated concentrations in myelinated nerve fibres, axons and glial membranes (Naidoo and Pratt 1951, Wolfgram and Rose 1960, Torack and Barnett 1964). 5'-nucleotidase was characterised as a particulate enzyme in cytochemical studies by Pope et al. (1957). 5'-nucleotidase activity was found to be increased in glioblastomas, moderate in astrocytomas and slight activities were encountered in meningiomas. The activity was not changed in brain tumour tissue cultures.

The steady state of adenine nucleotides, creatine phosphate and lactate levels have been found to be lower in ependymoblastoma than in brain. There were, however, enormous variations in the concentration of ATP within the tumours. The regions closest to the blood supply displayed the highest concentrations, whereas viable regions more distant from the blood supply exhibited low ATP levels (Maker et al. 1969).

The guanine nucleotide content of brain is relatively high, that is 18–20% of all nucleotides as compared with the liver or muscle guanine nucleotides (2–3%) (Schmitz et al. 1954).

Guanosine triphosphate (GTP) was found to play a rôle as cofactor of the α-ketoglutarate oxidase in brain (Wollemann 1959). Heald (1957) observed, after brief stimulation of brain slices, an increase in the turnover of guanosine di- and triphosphate. A specific rôle is also attributed to GTP in protein synthesis at the ribosomal level (Lucas-Lenard and Lipmann 1967). In spite of the diverse rôle of guanine nucleotides in brain metabbolism, nothing is known about their function in brain tumours.

2. Pyrimidine and pyridine nucleotides

Among the pyrimidine nucleotides, cytidine triphosphate is known to play a rôle in brain lecithin, phosphatidylethanolamine, phosphatidylserine and diphosphoinositide synthesis (see page 89). The intermediate compounds formed were identified as cytidine diphosphate choline and cytidine diphosphate ethanolamine (Kennedy and Weiss 1956). Uridine nucleotides also participate in brain metabolism as the intermediates uridine diphosphateglucose and uridine diphosphategalactose in the reversible enzymic transformation of galactose to glucose. These compounds are involved in the formation of galactolipids, gangliosides and neuraminic acids (Burton 1960).

The biosynthesis of pyrimidine nucleotides proceeds from carbamylphosphate via orotic acid. Two enzymes forming carbamylphosphate from ammonia, carbon dioxide and ATP are known: synthetase I which requires ammonia for activity and synthetase II which requires glutamine. Brain contains synthetase I; rapidly growing tissues such as liver, spleen and tumours contain synthetase II. The difference between the enzymes is also reflected in their subcellular distribution. Synthetase I is particle-bound, synthetase II is in the supernatant. Highest activities were found in the fastest growing transplanted tumours.

Other enzymes of pyrimidine synthesis are present in neoplastic tissue in much higher concentrations than carbamylphosphate synthetase. For example, the enzyme catalysing the next step of pyrimidine synthesis, aspartate carbamyltransferase is present in a hundredfold concentration in hepatomas compared with brain (Ono et al. 1963), and is 2–4 times higher compared with normal liver (Calva et al. 1959). Therefore synthetase II seems to be the rate limiting enzyme for the synthesis of uridine nucleotides in tumours (Yip and Knox 1970). In view of the presence of synthetase I in normal brain, synthetase activity measurements also seem to be of importance in brain tumours. The nucleotides diphosphopyridine and triphosphopyridine nucleotide (NAD, NADP) play a prominent rôle in many dehydrogenases as hydrogen carriers. NADP differs in one phosphoric acid group from NAD, which is attached in the 2′ position as a monoester on the ribose moiety of the adenylic acid part of the molecule. The NAD concentration dominates in brain, as in liver, over NADH, whereas NADPH prevails over NADP, although the NADP nucleotide content of brain is rather small compared to liver (one-fifth to one tenth). Mitochondria contain NAD in the oxidised form. Two transhydrogenases are present in mitochondria, one catalyses the hydrogen transfer from NADPH to NAD, the other from NADH to NAD (Kaplan et al. 1953).

NAD is decomposed in brain by a microsomal enzyme called diphospho-pyridine nucleotidase, which catalyses the reaction forming an adenosine diphosphate-ribose-enzyme complex in the first step. The second type of diphosphopyridine nucleotidase which attacks the pyrophosphate group is not present in brain (Jacobson and Kaplan 1957a).

The NAD and NADP content of tumour mitochondria is generally lower than that of normal tissue (see page 80). No consistent data exist to indicate the reason for this phenomenon, since elevated diphosphopyridine nucleotidase activity in tumours has been excluded by Quastel and Zatman (1953).

3. Synthesis and function of nucleic acids

It is beyond the scope of our treatise to deal here in detail with the compli-cated mechanism of nucleic acid metabolism and related protein synthesis, even though it involves some of the outstanding scientific achievements of our century. Nucleic acid metabolism and function were first investigated in bacteria, viruses and phages, followed by research on haematopoetic cells, liver cells, gametes and embryonic tissues. Although brain research on nucleic acid metabolism and function is rapidly expanding owing to a growing interest in memory investigations, there is still controversy even on the distribution of nucleic acid components and their base sequence (Oesterle et al. 1970, Bondy and Roberts 1968, Dawson 1967, Balázs and Cocks 1967, Jacob et al. 1966, Mahler et al. 1966, Hydén and Lange 1965). Agreement of data was achieved on the presence of labile and stable mes-senger RNA of brain cells (Zomzely et al. 1968, Appel 1967). Both authors consider the possibility of a highly responsive mechanism in the labile mRNA for associating the synthesis of certain proteins with coding, storage and utilisation of biological information.

To recapitulate the main parts of the processing of genetic information starting from DNA toward protein synthesis, we refer to Figure 3.31. The transcription of the genetic code from DNA to messenger RNA proceeds in the cell nucleus—forming complementary mRNA from the appropriate DNA template—from ribonucleotide triphosphates in the presence of an enzyme called RNA polymerase. This process was found to be reversible in mouse leukaemia (Baltimore 1970) and Rous sarcoma-producing viruses (Temin and Mizutani 1970). The reverse reaction is achieved with a RNA-dependent DNA polymerase of the virus. Thus the virus RNA serves as a template for the DNA synthesis from the nucleotides of the host. It seems very likely that all RNA tumour viruses have such activities. Recently, RNA-dependent DNA polymerase was also isolated in virus-like particles from human milk (Schlom et al. 1971) and from human lymphoblasts of leukaemic patients (Gallo et al. 1970). Congenital lack of enzymes in tissue culture could be corrected by infecting human fibroblasts with transducing bacterial viruses (Merril et al. 1971).

The next step in protein synthesis is called translation which refers to the
initiation, elongation and termination steps in protein synthesis. The mRNA
and the aminoacyl-transfer RNA are bound to the A (acceptor) binding
site of the 30 or 40 S particles of the ribosomes. Then the aminoacyl-tRNA
is transferred by a peptidyltransferase to the P (peptidyl) binding site of
the 50 or 60 S particles. During this time the ribosome slips over the messenger RNA chain through a triplet codon distance. This process is also called
translocation. Meanwhile a new aminoacyl-tRNA is bound to the A site

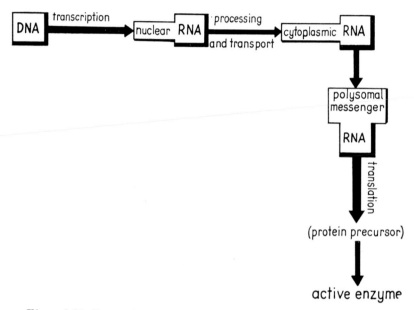

Figure 3.31. Processing of genetic information (Tomkins *et al.* 1969)

together with the next triplet codon of the mRNA. In this position a peptide
bond is formed between the free carboxyl group of the amino acid on the
P site and the amino group of the amino acid on the A site. After this the
whole process of translation starts again, and results in the newly formed
peptide chain on the P site continuing to elongate. This proceeds until
the last amino acid is released from the ribosomal particle. The association
and dissociation of the ribosomal particles in polysomal ribosomes is called
the ribosome cycle (Davis 1971). For the elongation other, different, protein
factors are necessary, for instance, the soluble elongation factors T
and G, which are connected with the newly elongated peptidyl-tRNA.
In *E. coli* the initiator of the protein synthesis in the presence of low Mg^{2+}
concentrations is a N-formylated-methionyl-tRNA in 70% of the investigated aminoacyl-tRNAs, together with the initiator code of the mRNA.
Several other initiating factors (F_1, F_2) and probably GTP are also required
(Lucas-Lenard and Lipmann 1967). In the absence of initiators, high Mg^{2+}

concentrations are necessary. The termination of protein synthesis is most likely initiated by the nonsense codon triplets (UAA, UAG) which do not code any amino acid. An enzymic release factor is probably also involved.

Apart from the cell nucleus, mitochondria also contain DNA, RNA and the complete apparatus for the synthesis of proteins. They are capable of reproducing themselves when the cell itself is not dividing. It has therefore been suggested that mitochondria were once free living organisms distantly related to present-day bacteria which were incorporated into larger cells and became endosymbiotic during evolution. A typical DNA molecule of animal cell mitochondria has a molecular weight 11.0×10^6, which is similar to the molecular weight of a smaller virus, or to a phage DNA containing several thousands of nucleotides. In comparison, the DNA of the nucleus of a bull sperm cell has a molecular veight of 3.2×10^9.

Bondy et al. (1970) recently discovered a very active histone-acetylating enzyme in brain tissue cell nuclei. It was supposed that acetylation of histones may result in the derepression of DNA and in the changed pattern of protein synthesis.

4. Inhibitors of nucleic acid metabolism

The increasing interest in the molecular mechanism of cell division and protein synthesis and the fatal consequences of tumour growth, stimulated research workers to find inhibitors of the different steps of nucleic acid metabolism. These efforts resulted in the search for various tumour growth inhibiting drugs, which are presently not fully efficient; however, some of them offer possibilities of relatively long remissions.

These drugs are partly synthetic and partly antibiotic (substances of natural origin) compounds. Some of them have already been referred to in the section on brain protein synthesis (see page 110), and after reviewing the steps of nucleic acid metabolism their site of attack will be more clear.

The inhibitors acting on nucleic acid synthesis may interfere with nucleotide metabolism, for example azaserine, which blocks purine synthesis and is an analogue of glutamine (Pitillo and Hunt 1967), or methotrexate (Timmis and Williams 1967), which interferes with nucleic acid synthesis by inhibiting the synthesis of tetrahydrofolate (the coenzyme of nucleotide synthesis). Base analogues, for instance 5-halogenated derivatives of uracil and uridine, also act as false substrates and may be incorporated into polynucleotides, disturbing the DNA template (Timmis and Williams 1967, Ács and Reich 1967).

Besides those interfering with nucleotide metabolism, drugs exerting a direct effect on nucleic acid synthesis were recently discovered. Among these rifamycin and streptovaricin act by inhibiting the activity of the RNA polymerase of bacteria and phages, having little or no effect on mammalian enzymes (Hartmann et al. 1968). This is very important in respect of the selective action of the drugs, and hope is offered for the specific inhibition of tumour virus RNA polymerase.

The third group of drugs interferes with nucleic acid synthesis by binding to the DNA template. This includes alkylating agents, for example, nitrogen and sulphur mustards (Lawley 1966) and the antibiotic mitomycin (Szybalski and Iyer 1967). They act bifunctionally by covalently binding with the DNA bases and by forming crosslinks between the DNA strands.

Other drugs form non-covalent complexes with DNA by distorting the structure and template activity. Among them the best known is actinomycin, which selectively inhibits transcription of the DNA template through the inhibition of RNA polymerase (Reich et al. 1964).

The last group of drugs binding to DNA include acridine (proflavine) (Blake and Peacocke 1968), phenanthridine (trypanocide ethidium) (Waring 1966), anthracycline (daunomycin, nogalamycin) (Ward et al. 1965) and chloroquine (O'Brien et al. 1966), which was known as an antimalarial drug. They act by intercalating their chromophore group between the adjacent base-pairs of the double helix of DNA (Lerman 1963).

Peptide bond formation at the ribosomal level (see also protein synthesis) is also inhibited by several antibiotics; of these puromycin has been most investigated. The chemical structure of puromycin is similar to the end structure of aminoacyl-tRNA. Puromycin is capable of replacing the aminoacyl adenosine moiety of the tRNA and therefore acts as a competitive substrate for peptide synthesis. A peptide bond is formed between the α-amino group of puromycin and the C-terminal end of a formyl-methionyl-peptidyl group. The product of the reaction, peptidyl-puromycin, is unable to take part in the next step of protein synthesis. Puromycin acts only on the 50 S or 60 S ribosome particles.

Among the antibiotics frequently used, chloramphenicol, certain macrolides (spiramycin, carbomycin, erythromycin, oleandomycin), streptogramin A and B, lincomycin and sparsomycin also act on the 50S particles of prokaryotes. Only puromycin and sparsomycin act on the 60S particles of eukaryotes together with the cycloheximide group, which, however, does not bind to the 50S particles. 30S and 40S particles are attacked by the tetracycline group, by edeine and polydextran sulphates, whereas the streptomycin group interferes only with the function of 30 S particles of the prokaryotes (Vazquez et al. 1970).

From the above enumeration it is evident that the inhibition of brain protein synthesis is only effective when drugs acting on 60 S or 40 S particles are used. In chemotherapy, however, the only drugs which can act selectively are those which inhibit the function of the 30 S or 50 S particles of bacterial origin without altering the protein synthesis of the host. Problems of selective tumour chemotherapy, supposing a viral origin, may be solved only on the level of specific inhibitors of viral RNA-dependent DNA polymerase.

5. Decomposition of nucleic acid

Two enzymes of nucleic acid catabolism are important in brain tumour investigations: deoxyribonuclease and ribonuclease. Deoxyribonuclease forms oligonucleotides from DNA which are further metabolised by specific phosphatases. Kunitz (1948) crystallised deoxyribonuclease from beef pancreas, and showed its pH optimum to be about seven, whereas the pH optimum of deoxyribonuclease from spleen, thymus, liver, intestinal mucosa and heart is about five (Koszalka *et al.* 1959). The enzyme from the pancreas is activated by bivalent cations (Mg^{2+}, Mn^{2+}, Co^{2+}) and inhibited by magnesium complexing compounds (citrate, arsenate, fluoride, EDTA). The second enzyme is activated by low concentrations of Mg^{2+}, while higher concentrations are inhibitory (Shack 1957). The two types of deoxyribonuclease (pancreas and spleen) were identified by disc electrophoresis (Ressler *et al.* 1966). Deoxyribonuclease I has a molecular weight of 30 700, splits oligonucleotides with phosphoryl groups in the 5' position and is inhibited by hydroxybiphenyls (Gottesfeld *et al.* 1971).

More information is available on ribonuclease. This is a phosphodiesterase which specifically splits the 3'phosphate bond from a pyrimidine nucleotide residue of RNA, with the intermediate formation of a pyrimidine cyclic phosphate. The enzymic action results in mixtures of mono- and oligonucleotides, according to the site of pyrimidine nucleotides in the RNA chain. Ribonuclease from pancreas was first obtained in a crystalline form by Kunitz (1940). The separation of the recrystallised bovine pancreatic ribonuclease into two active forms was one of the first demonstrations of heterogeneity in a crystalline enzyme (Martin and Porter 1951). The two forms, called A and B resemble each other very closely (Tanford and Hauenstein 1956). Ribonuclease was the first enzyme to have its primary structure described, mainly by Hirs *et al.* (1960) and Spackman *et al.* (1960). It consists of one hundred and twenty-four amino acids. The tertiary structure of bovine pancreas ribonuclease was also determined (Kartha *et al.* 1967). Kinetic studies showed that the histidine residues (twelve and one hundred and nineteen) are involved in the catalytic action. The three-dimensional structure is stabilised by four SH bridges between eight cysteine molecules in the ribonuclease (26–84; 40–97; 58–110; 65–72). They are reduced by urea treatment which causes changes in the tertiary conformation and a reversible loss in enzyme activity. The acid deoxyribonuclease and ribonuclease are both lysosome-bound enzymes in brain tissue as demonstrated by Koenig *et al.* (1964). Vorbrodt (1961) reported that acid ribonuclease was present in both lysosomes and nuclei of a variety of cells. Purified pancreas ribonuclease was first applied by Brachet (1940) to demonstrate that the Nissl granules contain RNA.

6. Neoplastic changes in nucleic acid metabolism

Investigations on the nucleic acid metabolism of brain tumours are very scarce in comparison with other tumour investigations. The transfer and ribosomal RNA in brain tumours has been shown to differ qualitatively from normal brain. The ratio of the methylated bases in the tRNA fraction increases proportionately with malignancy when compared with the normal brain and the ribosomal pattern of the 18 S and 28 S particles. The activity of the RNA synthetase is different in brain tumours (Viale *et al.* 1969, Viale and Kroh 1971, Wender *et al.* 1971). Transfer RNA methylase activity also increased and changed in specificity in cancer and various other tumours (Craddock 1970) and altered tRNA was detected in Morris hepatomas (Volkers and Taylor 1971).

Deoxyribonuclease and ribonuclease were investigated in the cystic fluid of brain tumours. Deoxyribonuclease was found to be particularly active in the cystic fluid of the more undifferentiated tumours (Spiegel-Adolf and Wycis 1954, 1957). Deoxyribonuclease and ribonuclease activities have been found to decrease in rat liver tumours with neoplastic transformation (De Lamirande *et al.* 1961). A decrease of ribonuclease activity was also found in hyperplastic cells by Amano and Daoust (1961) and Vorbrodt (1961).

Weber and Lea (1965) found that a gradual increase in biosynthesis and a decrease in the catabolism of nucleic acids could be correlated with an increase in growth rate. This was measured as an increase of DNA synthesis reflected by enhanced thymidine-2-^{14}C incorporation and increased formate incorporation into DNA and RNA, while labelled adenine incorporation into DNA and RNA was high in all tumours. DNA levels correlated with tumour growth but RNA levels did not. These values are somewhat similar to the DNA content of the glioma group as described by Heller and Elliott (1954) (see page 38) and seem to contradict the results of Spiegel-Adolf and Wycis (1957). A decreased DNA and RNA catabolism, reflected in decreased uracil and thymine reductase, xanthine oxidase and uricase activities, was also encountered by Weber and Lea (1965). The DNA and RNA contents of tumour cells were observed to change in parallel and were approximately proportional to the chromosome number. Tetraploid cells of ascites, lymphomas and carcinoma of mice were found to be twice that of adjacent diploid cells (Kit 1960). Laird and Barton (1956) observed that the concentration of RNA in tumours was higher in the nuclear fractions of tumour cells compared with normal cells. Kit (1960) did not observe significant differences between the DNA of normal tissues or tumours with respect to base composition. Sporn (1971) suggested that the primary lesion in malignant tumours is not in the DNA itself but is a permanent molecular lesion in the processing of nuclear RNA.

Polyribosomes of normal liver and experimental hepatomas differ in their abnormally high monomer and dimer peaks and the presence of an X component (Webb and Potter 1966) which represents a reserve pool for forming active polyribosomes. Webb and Morris (1969) suggested that the abnormal monomer–dimer peak in hepatomas may be due to a deficiency of the initiating factors. Griffin (1964) reported that the first peak of phenyl-alanyl-tRNA in Novikoff ascites tumour cells was absent and the second peak was displaced, in contrast to the liver pattern. Labile messenger RNA templates were observed by Greengard and Smith (1963) in hepatoma. The authors concluded that altered template stability resulting from changes in the molecular pattern of the cellular membrane surface could be the mechanism of the malignant transformation. The formation of labile messenger RNA was also observed in brain, where it was attributed with a function in the coding of information (Zomzely *et al.* 1968) (see page 117).

Changes in Nucleotide and Nucleic Acid Metabolism
in Brain Tumours

Enzyme activity	Type of tumour			
	GL	GB	AC	MG
Creatine kinase	±[1]			
Myokinase	±[1]			
5-Nucleotidase		+[2]	+[2]	−[2]
Ribonuclease	+[3]			
Deoxyribonuclease	+[4]			

+ = increased; − = decreased; ± = unchanged.
[1] Lehrer (1962), [2] Matakas (1969), [3] Spiegel-Adolf and Wycis
(1954), [4] Spiegel-Adolf and Wycis (1957).

3.10. HYDROLYTIC ENZYMES

1. Lysosomal enzymes

In the last part of this treatise on brain tumour metabolism, several enzymes are reviewed which have a catabolic function and were discovered mainly in lysosomes. Lysosomes are cytoplasmic cell particles derived from the Golgi endoplasmic reticulum. They have in common a high content of acid hydrolytic enzymes.

De Duve *et al.* (1955), De Duve (1959) described the lysosome as an inert osmotic sac which is limited by an impermeable lipoprotein membrane that restricts the substrate accessibility to the enclosed hydrolytic enzymes. The membrane is stabilised by glucocorticoids, which may owe some of their protective effects against cell injury to their ability to strengthen the membrane of lysosomes against disruption. Neural lysosomes also contain acid hydrolases and a matrix which seems to consist of protein associated lipids (Koenig *et al.* 1964). Lysosomes show, after acridine orange staining, a bright orange fluorescence (Dingle and Barrett 1960).

The function of lysosomes in the cell consists of intra- and extracellular digestion; heterophagic functions are the defence reaction against toxins, bacteria, viruses and other microorganisms. An autophagic function is also attributed to lysosomes: this consists of self digestion under certain pathological conditions. In brain tumours lysosomes have been identified by histochemical, electron-microscopic and differential centrifugation methods (Figure 3.32) (Wollemann *et al.* 1965, Wollemann 1967, Sutton and Becker 1969). Sutton and Becker (1969) demonstrated the presence of lysosomes in increased numbers in the cytoplasm of neoplastic cells as compared with resting and reactive astrocytes. They also exploited the heterophagic activity of lysosomes to incorporate labelled proteins and peroxidase which entered the cell by the pinocytosis and were readily taken into the lysosomes of the tumour cells. The authors consider it possible to introduce into tumour cells cytotoxic groups bound to protein carriers, using this mechanism.

Increased lysosomal activity was observed in cells of microglial origin and macrophages around necrotic parts; also in giant tumour cells, in cells of glioblastomas of astrocytic origin and in the form of coarse and fine gran-

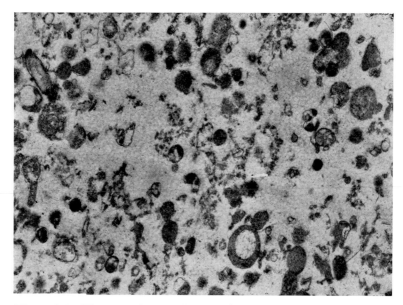

Figure 3.32. Electron-micrograph of the lysosome-enriched cell fraction from glioblastoma multiforme No. 258, prepared according to Stahl *et al.* (1963). Enlargement 18 000 diameters

ules in meningiomas scattered in the cytoplasm of round cells, presumably histiocytes. Thus glioma cells are characterized by increased lysosomal enzyme activities. These are most probably due to autolytic reactions of the tumour cells or in the case of immigrated macrophages and microglial cells, heterophagy occurs as a defence reaction of the host against the invasion of tumour cells.

Among hydrolases in general are classified those enzymes which split different groups of chemical compounds (esters, peptides, glycosides) in the presence of water

$$S + H_2O \xrightarrow{E} P_1H + P_2OH$$

where s = Substrate

 e = Enzyme

 P_1 and P_2 = products (acids, alcohols or amines)

Some of these enzymes have been mentioned in sections 3.8.4 (glutaminase, asparaginase, peptidase and proteinase) and 3.9.1–6 (nucleotidase, ribonuclease, adenosinetriphosphatase and deoxyribonuclease). In the following sections, the hydrolases, which are localised partly in the lysosomes and play an important rôle in brain tumour catabolism, will be considered; these are the phosphatases, esterases, β-glucuronidase and β-galactosidase.

2. Phosphatases

Two phosphomonoesterases were prominent in the history of brain tumours: alkaline and acid phosphatase. Alkaline phosphatase has a pH optimum around 9 and splits phosphoric acid esters of aliphatic alcohols (glycerophosphate), phenols (phenylphosphates), cyclic alcohols (naphthylphosphates, phenolphthalein phosphate), nucleoside phosphates and inorganic pyrophosphate. It is competitively inhibited by inorganic phosphate or arsenate. Alkaline phosphatase was purified from intestinal phosphatase and Morton (1955) established for it a molecular weight of 60 000. In brain it was purified from microsomes and ribosomes of the cortex of goats. It showed a higher activity with nucleoside phosphates than with sugar monophosphates (Saraswathi and Bachhawat 1966). In the nervous system, it is concentrated mainly in the capillary and vascular endothelium and the arachnoid and pial endothelium. The activity of grey matter was twice that of white matter.

Alkaline phosphatase occurs in multiple molecular forms. Robinson and Pierce (1964) demonstrated that three of the four alkaline phosphatase isoenzymes in man contained terminal neuraminic acid. The isoenzymes possibly differ in their carbohydrate content. β-lipoproteins of serum and tissues also displayed alkaline phosphatase activity (Moss and King 1962). Serum alkaline phosphatase originates predominantly from liver and not from bones as previously supposed. This was shown by starch gel isoenzyme studies (Hodson et al. 1962). Two alkaline phosphatase isoenzymes have been separated from sheep brain with different substrate affinities and localisation (Saraswathi and Bachhawat 1966) (Figure 3.33).

Brain tumour enzyme histochemistry started in 1942 with the demonstration of alkaline phosphatase activity in meningiomas by Landow. This was followed by a series of other publications on the alkaline phosphatase activity of brain tumours, mainly in meningiomas (Friede 1956, Büttger et al. 1957, Feigen and Wolf 1958, Kirsch 1963, Udvarhelyi et al.

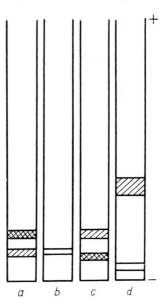

Figure 3.33. Alkaline phosphatase isoenzymes demonstrated according to Gomori (1952), thalamus of twenty-six weeks old human embryonic brain No. 324 (*a*), mixed glioma No. 319 tumour(*b*) and tumour surrouning tissue (*c*), neurinoma No. 306 (*d*)

1962, O'Connor *et al.* 1963). Alkaline phosphatase activity was usually higher in meningiomas than in gliomas, apart from ependymomas, and seemed to be related to the vascularity of the tumours. According to Meyer-Ruge (1966) glioblastoma multiforme revealed no capillary alkaline phosphatase activity. This indicates a loss of function of the blood-brain barrier, and is probably the cause of necrosis and bleeding inside the tumour. Alkaline phosphatase activity was higher in other gliomas with marked vascularity, but neuroglia exhibited low activity. The most active parts in meningiomas were the capillary endothelia and there was a definite tendency for increased activity in whorls and around psammome bodies. These results were obtained by the diazonium method (Menten *et al.* 1944). Previous investigations carried out with the calcium phosphate method of Gomori (1939) also showed activity in the cell nuclei and membranes.

Osske *et al.* (1968) differentiated between three types of meningiomas according to their alkaline phosphatase activity. In the first type the activity was present only in the blood vessel walls, in the second only in the cytoplasm of the tumour cells and in the third type the activity was enhanced at both sites. Plasma activity exhibited very faint staining with naphthylphosphates but only with β-glycerophosphates; they therefore supposed the presence of two different isoenzymes. Fischer and Müller (1970) demonstrated that the alkaline phosphatase activity of tumour cells is identical to the activity of the enzymes of the leptomeninx and choroid plexus in pH optimum, K_m, heat stability, inhibition by phenylalanine, relative activity towards different substrates and electrophoresis in agar and starch gel. Reactive astrocytes showed no activity. They supposed that the loss of enzyme activity in other meningioma tumour cells was an enzyme deletion taking place in the course of tumour progression and was a sign of an increasing degree of malignancy. The authors explained generally the appearance of new types of isoenzymes by a genetic derepression in tumours, but did not consider the possibility of new DNA synthesis by RNA containing viruses (Temin and Mizutani 1970). Experimentally induced brain tumours, as demonstrated by Kirsch (1963), displayed similar low alkaline phosphatase activities to human brain tumours (anaplastic gliomas and sarcomas), whereas well differentiated ependymomas showed high activities.

Müller and Nasu (1960, 1962) demonstrated in neurinomas that the alkaline phosphatase activity was present only in blood vessel walls. Samorajski and McCloud (1961) concluded that an elevated enzyme activity occurs with the increase in permeability of blood vessels in oedema, meningioma and meningo-encephalomyelitis. According to Kreuzberg *et al.* (1967) and Matakas (1969) the alkaline phosphatase activity was increased in tissue cultures of all the tumours investigated except oligodendrogliomas and primary brain sarcomas. Cumings (1962) observed an increase in alkaline phosphatase activity in the microsomal fraction of oedematous white matter. In brain tumour cysts no alkaline phosphatase activity was recovered (Szliwovski and Cumings 1961). The histochemical alkaline phosphatase reaction was also widely used in the diagnosis of different neoplasms. Thus Gomori (1955) was able to differentiate between Ewing's tumour and neuroblastoma, because the latter showed a negative reaction. Intense activity was found in adenocarcinomas of the small intestine and in adrenal cortical tumours.

Changes in the alkaline and acid phosphatase activities in cystic fluid were not parallel with the malignancy of the brain tumours, in contrast to the lactic dehydrogenase and phosphohexose isomerase activities (Buckell and Robertson 1965).

The demonstration of alkaline phosphatase isoenzymes in the serum of patients with secondary liver tumours, Paget's disease, and osteoplastic bone tumours, disclosed isoenzymes with abnormal motilities in agar gel electrophoresis (Haije and de Jong 1963).

In obvious contrast to the many observations dealing with the alkaline phosphatase activity of tumours are the limited data on the physiological or pathological rôle of this enzyme. None of the applied substrates can be regarded as native to the organism. The authors are reduced to conjectures based on the physiological localisation in the blood vessel wall, the lepto-meninx and choroid plexus, that it might play a rôle in the transport of some phosphate esters across the blood brain barrier. This is supported by the high alkaline phosphatase activity in cases of permeability increase in oedema and in meningo-encephalomyelitis (Samorajski and McCloud 1961). Another suggestion is that in the presence of suitable phosphate receptors alkaline phosphatase might act as a transphosphorylase, which offers new functional aspects (Cohen 1970).

Acid phosphatase is a lysosomal enzyme which has a pH optimum of 4–6 in the different tissues. It is a monophosphoesterase similar to alkaline phosphatase, with similar substrates and inhibitors. However, acid phos-phatase is not activated by Mg^{2+} ions, in contrast to alkaline phosphatase. Acid phosphatase is present in the lysosomes of neurones and neuroglia according to several authors (Lazarus et al. 1962, Becker et al. 1960). Acid phosphatase also occurs in multiple forms. Anderson and Song (1962) found 3–4 bands in rat brain and Barron (1963) two bands in human brain. The K_m of the isoenzymes was, however, different, unlike the alkaline phosphat-ase isoenzymes. Sur et al. (1962) using specific inhibitors (ethanol, L-tartarate, formaldehyde) established differences between the isoenzymes of different organs (prostate, liver, erythrocytes). Using buffers below pH 7.0, the electrophoretic separation was more specific and up to thirteen bands could be revealed from the prostatic enzyme (Lundin and Allison 1966). Treat-ment of acid phosphatase from the human prostate gland with neuramin-idase abolishes its electrophoretic heterogeneity but does not inhibit its enzyme activity (Ostrowski et al. 1970).

Acid phosphatase activity in brain tumours was first investigated by histo-chemical methods mainly in meningiomas (Wolf et al. 1943, Büttger et al. 1957, Anderson and Song 1962). In contrast to alkaline phosphatase activity, no specifically increased reactions were observed which correlated directly or inversely with malignancy. Acid phosphatase activity was increased in different reactive glial cells of gemistocytic and microglial origin, where it was localised in the form of coarse granules in the lysosomes (Figure 3.34). In the neurinomas, the activity in the cells of the Antoni (1920) B zones was localised in large granules whereas in the cells of the Antoni A zones

multiple fine granules occurred. The increased lysosomal activity in the B
zone should be regarded as a phagocytic reaction of the Schwann cells
(Wollemann *et al.* 1965, Wollemann 1970, Sutton and Becker 1969). Müller
and Nasu (1960) observed a similar patchy distribution in neurinomas,
which was localised in the lipopigment granules. Lipopigments are possibly
produced by the transformation of lysosomes.

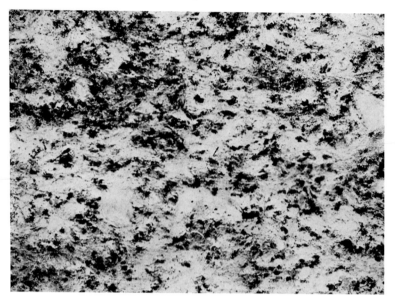

Figure 3.34. Acid phosphatase activity in glioblastoma No. 194. Histochemical slide stained according to Burstone (1958). Intense activity
in numerous microglial cells distributed diffusely throughout an extensive zone of necrosis. Magnification 130×

Increased acid phosphatase activity was demonstrated in a variety of
tumours (hepatoma, carcinomas) by biochemical (Greenstein and Thompson
1943) and histochemical methods (Gomori 1955). Reiner *et al.* (1957)
observed that the acid phosphatase activity of a ganglioneurinoma was
concentrated in a group of intensely stained 'ganglion cells'. Gerhardt *et al.*
(1963) localised the acid phosphatase activity in brain tumours to the α
and β-globulins. Activity in the prealbumin region was observed in neurinomas. In meningiomas intense activity in the α-globulin fraction was also
encountered. Acid phosphatase activity was demonstrated by starch gel
electrophoresis in two equally distributed isoenzymes. In meningiomas and
glioblastomas two additional bands migrating toward the cathode and one
toward the anode were also encountered (Wollemann *et al.* 1965, Wollemann
1970) (see Table IX). Grundig *et al.* (1965) and Goldberg *et al.* (1966) investigated the serum phosphatase isoenzymes in patients with Gaucher's disease,
prostatic carcinoma and multiple myeloma. Some cases exhibited more
isoenzymes than observed in normal sera.

The rôle of acid phosphatase activity is clearer than that of alkaline phosphatase owing to its lysosomal localisation, although the question of its physiological substrate still remains open.

TABLE IX

Distribution of acid phosphatase activity in human brain tumours on starch gel electrophoresis. (Figures represent percentage contribution of each band to the activity)

Tumour No.	Band No.							
	+	3	2	1	0	1	2	—
Glioblastoma								
No. 359		14	36	50		—	—	
No. 195		—	43	33		15	9	
Meningioma (end.)								
No. 432		26	74	—		—	—	
No. 197		48	10	24		14	4	
Meningioma (fibr.)								
No. 166		—	80	20		—	—	
Metastatic carcinoma								
No. 90		—	15	85		—	—	
Neurinoma								
No. 169		19	81	—		—	—	
No. 47		23	77	—		—	—	

3. Esterases

After phosphatases, the next very important group of hydrolase enzymes are the esterases. According to Augustinsson (1958, 1961) the esterases include three groups of enzymes: two nonspecific esterases (aromatic- and aliphatic- or arylesterases and aliesterases) and a specific esterase, cholinesterase. The characteristics of the three groups are somewhat overlapping. Aliphatic esters of acetate and butyrate are hydrolysed by aliesterases, whereas arylesterases preferentially hydrolyse only aromatic esters (phenyl-esters of acetate or butyrate). Cholinesters are specifically hydrolysed by the cholinesterases (Figure 3.38). Another classification of esterases is given by Aldridge (1954), who differentiates between A and B types of esterases apart from cholinesterases. Esterase A is identical with aromatic esterase and B with aliesterase. The C type esterase splits carboxylic acid esters, but it is not inhibited by DFP (diisopropylfluorophosphate) nor does it hydrolyse it (Bergmann et al. 1957).

Plasma cholinesterase was first measured in equine sera by Stedman and Stedman (1935). Later Alles and Hawes (1940) and Mendel and Rudney (1949) established that two different cholinesterases are present in the organism, one which hydrolyses acetylcholine more readily, the other which was more effective with choline esters of longer chain length, such as butyrylcholine or with aromatic cholinesters. Acetylcholinesterase is localised in

9

high concentrations in nervous and muscle tissue and in erythrocytes. Butyrylcholinesterase is present in serum, liver, intestine and in the white matter of brain. Results on the localisation of cholinesterases in the nervous system are not in complete agreement. The acetylcholinesterase activity is highest in the caudate nucleus, followed by the lentiform nucleus and the cerebellar hemispheres (Burgen and Chipman 1951), whereas the white matter contains significantly more pseudocholinesterase than the grey matter (Ord and Thompson 1952, Foldes *et al*. 1962). Histochemical methods revealed a localisation of acetylcholinesterase in the Nissl granules (Fukada and Koelle 1959), activity was also present in the perikaryon, axons and dendrites of neurones (Koelle 1954, 1955). Electron-microscopic investigations in frog sympathetic and dorsal root ganglia and rat brain revealed acetylcholinesterase activity on the inner surface of the endoplasmic reticulum, nuclear envelope, subsurface cisternae and agranular reticulum of the perikaryon and axon (Torack and Barnett 1962, Brzin *et al*. 1966). After ultracentrifugation of cell particles acetylcholinesterase was localised in the microsomal and mitochondrial cell fractions (Holmstedt and Toschi 1959, Giacobini 1960). Density gradient centrifugation showed that acetylcholinesterase is associated with the membrane of the nerve-endings (De Robertis 1963). Considerable activities were also recovered in the supernatant. The localisation of acetylcholine hydrolysing enzymes differed from that of the acetylcholine synthesising enzyme. Thus choline acetylase (choline-O-acetyltransferase), which synthesises acetylcholine from choline and acetyl-CoA is located, according the majority of authors, in the synaptic vesicles (Hebb and Whittaker 1958, De Robertis 1963), but Michaelson (1967) recovered choline-acetyltransferase only in the supernatant. In mouse neuroblastoma cell cultures, an inverse relationship was observed for the regulation of choline acetylase and thymidylate synthetase. When cell division is restricted in confluent cultures choline acetylase activity is high and thymidylate synthetase activity is low, the opposite result was observed when the cells were growing rapidly (Rosenberg *et al*. 1971).

Butyrylcholinesterase was localised by histochemical methods in astrocytes and other glial cells and in the smooth muscle of blood vessels. Using the subcellular fractionation method (Holmstedt and Toschi 1959), the activity was found to be concentrated in the supernatant and microsomal fractions of rat brain (Parmar *et al*. 1961). Aldridge and Johnson (1959) reported that nonspecific cholinesterase is concentrated in the nuclear fraction. The different results are probably due to the different animal species and methods used in the experiments. The localisation of the enzymes in the Nissl substance, microsomes, endoplasmic reticulum and lysosomes is closely related and corresponds to the applied histochemical or differential centrifugation methods.

Acetylcholinesterase was crystallised from the electric tissue of *Electrophorus electricus* by Leuzinger and Baker (1967), Leuzinger *et al*. (1969), who found its molecular weight to be 260 000. It is a glycoprotein containing glucosamines and galactosamines. The enzyme has a dimeric hybrid structure with two types of polypeptide chains and consists of four subunits with a molecular weight of 64 000.

Butyrylcholinesterase was purified from serum and liver. It was obtained in a homogeneous form from human serum by Das and Liddel (1970). Its molecular weight is 366 000. Svensmark (1963) also purified human liver cholinesterase and identified fraction II as serum cholinesterase. The cholinesterase fraction I differed from serum cholinesterase in that it contained no sialic acids. Fraction I is regarded as a precursor of serum cholinesterase. Neuraminidase treatment of serum cholinesterase splits the sialic acids and results in a change of electrophoretic mobility without loss of enzyme activity (Svensmark and Kristensen 1963).

The main difference between the two types of cholinesterases is reflected in their substrate specificity. Acetylcholinesterase hydrolyses acetylcholine at an optimal rate of 3×10^{-3} K_m in the brain and is inhibited by an excess of substrate. Acetyl-β-methylcholine is hydrolysed only by acetylcholinesterase, whereas butyrylcholinesterase is inactive against it and is not inhibited by high concentrations of acetylcholine substrate. The K_m for acetylcholine using acetylcholinesterase from beef erythrocytes and equine serum cholinesterase was 1.9×10^{-4} and 1.5×10^{-3} respectively, indicating a ten times higher affinity of acetylcholine to acetylcholinesterase than to butyrylcholinesterase (Zech 1969). Other cholinesters, such as propionylcholine or benzoylcholine, are hydrolysed only by butyrylcholinesterase (Mendel and Rudney 1943).

Specific inhibitors are also used to differentiate between acetylcholinesterase and butyrylcholinesterase. These are alkylphosphates (DFP, TEPP, sarin, iso-OMPA and parathion), which act by phosphorylating the hydroxyl group of serine in the active centre of serum cholinesterase, which is ten times more sensitive to alkylphosphate inhibition than acetylcholinesterase. This phosphorylation can be reversed by the addition of pyridine-2-aldoxime methiodide (Wilson and Ginsburg 1955). Among other inhibitors 62C47, mytelase and BW 284C51 are used as specific inhibitors of acetylcholinesterase, and Ro 2–0683 and diethazine as inhibitors of butyrylcholinesterase. Some of the alkylphosphate inhibitors (DFP, parathion) also inhibit aliphatic esterase activity. Eserine inhibits both types of cholinesterases, but none of the different esterases.

According to the original conception of Bergman et al. (1950) cholinesterase has two substrate binding groups on the active surface: one anionic, which binds the quaternary nitrogen of acetylcholine, and one esteric at a distance of 5 Å, which binds the carbonyl group of the ester bond. The anionic site is represented by glutamic and aspartic acids, whereas serine and histidine are present at the esteric site (Jansz et al. 1959). According to Krupka (1966, 1967) the hydrolysis of acetylcholine proceeds in two steps. First, the enzyme is acetylated at the serine site and the quaternary nitrogen is bound to the anionic site. In the second step the enzyme is deacetylated after the hydrolysis of the substrate.

The multiplicity of the two cholinesterases was also demonstrated with electrophoretic methods by different authors. Serum cholinesterase was resolved into several fractions by electrophoresis according to the applied method by Pinter (1957), Dubbs et al. (1960), Bernsohn et al. (1961), Hess et al. (1963a) and Juul (1968) (Figure 3.35).

9*

According to La Motta *et al.* (1968) the heterogeneity of serum cholinesterase cannot be completely explained by assuming polymer forms for the enzyme, although the isoenzymes are interconvertible.

It was possible to determine the molecular weights of the different human serum cholinesterase isoenzymes by density gradient ultracentrifugation. The results are as follows: CHE_1, 82 000; CHE_2, 110 000; CHE_3, 170 000; CHE_4, 200 000; CHE_5, 260 000 (La Motta *et al.* 1970). Gaffney (1968) suggested that the more anionic components of the enzyme contain various amounts of sialic acids, whereas the less anionic forms may be explained by polymerisation. In some sera of low enzyme activity an atypical cholinesterase activity was established with different inhibitory and hydrolytic capacities (Kalow and Staron 1957). The low cholinesterase activity is genetically determined by two codominant allelic genes (Lehmann and Ryan 1956, Lehmann and Silk 1964). Only slight differences from normal cholinesterase were observed in the electrophoretic mobilities of the isoenzymes of the atypical cholinesterase (Kalow and Davies 1959). Selectively weak, fast moving isoenzymes have been demonstrated by several authors (Hodgkin *et al.* 1965, Brody *et al.* 1965).

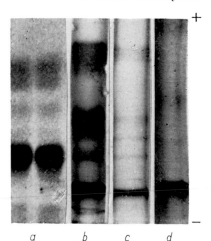

Figure 3.35. Esterase and cholinesterase isoenzymes from human sera stained according to Nachlas *et al.* (1952) demonstrated on starch gel (*a*) and disc gel (*b, c, d*); normal human sera (*a*) (*c*), plasmocytoma No. 22 (*b*) and hypophysis adenoma No. 31 (*d*). Note the increase of all fractions in (*b*) and the selective increase of choinesterase in (*d*)

Multiple forms of acetylcholinesterase from nervous tissue have also been shown (Bernsohn *et al.* 1962). Using acetylthiocholine and butyrylthiocholine as substrate, three isoenzymes have been demonstrated from human brain caudate nucleus and putamen. Two acetylcholinesterase isoenzymes did not differ in pH optimum, K_m values and inhibition with eserine, mytelase and DFP (Bernsohn *et al.* 1962). Wollemann *et al.* (1965), Wollemann (1967) demonstrated three isoenzymes using butyrylthiocholine and acetylthiocholine as substrate, but only two isoenzymes with acetyl-β-methylthiocholine were demonstrated in human corpus striatum, cerebellum, grey matter of cortex and subcortical white matter (Figures 3.36*a, b*).

Investigations on the cholinesterase activity of brain tumours were first carried out by Youngstrom *et al.* (1941). Using acetylcholine as substrate they revealed high activities in gliomas, especially astrocytomas and glioblastomas. Low activities were encountered in meningiomas, spongioblastomas and metastatic carcinoma. Bülbring *et al.* (1953) investigated eight gliomas, one neurinoma and three meningiomas using acetylcholine, butyrylcholine and acetyl-β-methylcholine as substrate, and obtained high butyryl-

Acetylcholine Metabolism

Substrate	Enzyme	Coenzyme	Inhibitor	Product	Receptor inhibitor
1. acetate	acetylkinase	CoA, ATP		acetyl CoA	decamethonium succinylcholine
2. acetyl CoA + choline	cholineacetylase		hemicholine	acetylcholine	curare (motor endplate) atropine (ganglia) hexamethonium
3. acetylcholine	cholinesterase		organic P: DFP, TEPP, OMPA sarine, tabun, parathion, paraoxon quaternary $-$ NH$_3^+$ neostigmine, mestinon, tensilon, mytelase	acetate, choline	nicotine (high doses) bungarotoxin

cholinesterase activities in gliomas. Acetylcholinesterase activity was
highest in the acoustic neurinoma. The lowest activities were encountered
in meningiomas. Cavanagh *et al.* (1954) also found high values of butyrylcholinesterase activity in twenty-one gliomas (glioblastoma, spongioblastoma, astrocytoma and oligodendroglioma). Lower activities were encountered in meningiomas and medulloblastomas, with one exception. The authors
concluded that the butyrylcholinesterase activity is associated with the
supportive glial cells rather than with cells of the conducting system and
that the vascular elements of the tumours do not contribute to any great
degree to the enzyme activities.

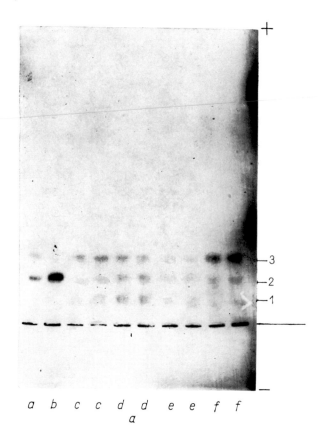

Figure 3.36a. Cholinesterase patterns of
supernatants of various areas of normal
human brain and brain tumours after starch
gel electrophoresis using butyrylthiocholine
as substrate according the method of Koelle
(1951). Meningioma No. 193 (*a*), glioblastoma
No. 411 (*b*), subcortical white matter (*c*),
cortical grey matter (*d*), cerebellar cortex (*e*),
caudate nucleus and putamen (*f*)

Wollemann and Zoltán (1962) reported acetyl- and butyrylcholinesterase activities in one hundred cases of brain tumours and fifty tumorous cysts. Butyrylcholinesterase activity was strongly enhanced in gliomas (twenty-eight glioblastomas, twenty-six astrocytomas, two oligodendrogliomas). Both types of cholinesterase were reduced in nine metastatic carcinomas, twenty-four meningiomas, four neurinomas and four craniopharyngeomas. The butyrylcholinesterase activity of the tumourous cysts was, in all investigated cases, higher than the acetylcholinesterase activity, irrespective of the

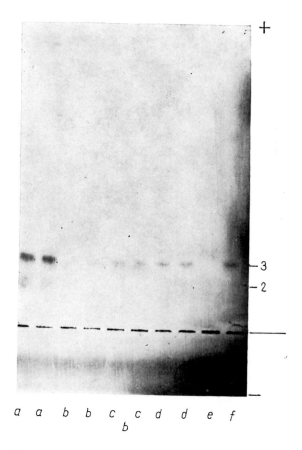

Figure 3.36b. Cholinesterase patterns of supernatants of various areas of normal human brain and brain tumours after starch gel electrophoresis using acetyl-β-methylthiocholine as substrate, according the method of Koelle (1951), caudate nucleus and putamen (*a*), cerebellar cortex (*b*), cortical grey matter (*c*), subcortical white matter (*d*), glioblastoma No. 411 (*e*), meningioma No. 193 (*f*)

tumour type (twenty glioblastomas, twenty-two astrocytomas, four cranio-pharyngeomas, four metastatic carcinomas) (see Table X). In investigations using differential centrifugation, the acetylcholinesterase activity was diminished in the particulate fraction of all types of the tumours examined (glioblastoma, meningioma, astrocytoma and metastatic carcinoma) compared with normal grey matter. The butyrylcholinesterase activity in

TABLE X

Cholinesterase activities of brain tumours and cysts.
Results are expressed as μg substrate hydrolysed/mg protein/hour ($\bar{x} \pm \delta$)

Sample	No. of samples examined	ACH	BuCH	MeCH
Tumours				
Glioblastoma	28	171.7 ± 8.7	355.6 ± 20.7	29.9 ± 4.4
Astrocytoma	26	242.3 ± 20.6	456.7 ± 22.5	35.7 ± 7.3
Meningioma	24	53.3 ± 4.5	27.3 ± 2.3	30.1 ± 2.7
Metastatic carcinoma	9	55.3 ± 5.7	113.1 ± 9.2	18.1 ± 2.8
White matter	3	102.0 ± 20.4	185.0 ± 13.2	—
Grey matter	8	563.4 ± 58.0	283.9 ± 18.0	365.5 ± 25.9
Cysts				
Glioblastoma multiforme	20	142.5 ± 26.0	340.2 ± 32.3	2.1 ± 0.8
Astrocytoma	22	156.2 ± 14.1	371.2 ± 18.6	1.0 ± 0.5
Normal serum	4	400.5 ± 31.3	688.5 ± 18.4	—

δ = Standard deviation.

gliomas was enhanced in all fractions, but the highest increase was encountered in the microsomal fraction as compared with normal white matter (Wollemann and Zoltán 1962, Wollemann et al. 1969, Wollemann 1970).

Perria et al. (1964) used acetylthiocholine and butyrylthiocholine as substrate to measure the cholinesterase activity of brain tumours. The values obtained for butyrylthiocholine hydrolysis in the manometric technique were higher in astrocytomas and glioblastomas than for the acetylthiocholine hydrolysis. With histochemical methods, acetylcholinesterase activity was not demonstrated in tissue slides and cultures of brain tumours (Kreuzberg and Gullotta 1967, Augusti-Tocco and Sato 1969) except in neuroblastomas (Wollemann et al. 1965, Wollemann 1970, Matakas 1969). In cultured neuroblastoma cells the induction of acetylcholinesterase was observed after adding nucleotides (Kates et al. 1971).

While investigating the distribution of the acetylcholinesterase and butyrylcholinesterase isoenzymes in brain tumours, the following changes were encountered when compared with normal brain tissue: The first cathodal band in starch gel electrophoresis, with butyrylthiocholine or acetylthio-

choline as substrate, was consistently absent in gliomas, metastatic carcinomas and meningiomas, but was present in neurinomas and neuroblastomas. Band two, which is probably identical with serum cholinesterase, was
markedly increased in most of the tumours, compared with normal brain.
The anodal band three was absent in some of the glioblastomas (Figure 3.41,
Tables XI, XII). With acetyl-β-methylthiocholine as substrate in the starch

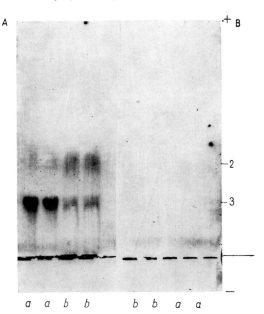

Figure 3.37. Cholinesterase patterns
of supernatants of brain tumours after starch gel electrophoresis, stained
with butyrylthiocholine. Glioblastoma
No. 174 (*a*), oligodendroglioma No.
150 (*b*). Side B is inhibited with 10^{-6} M
RO2-0683. Side A, control

gel electrophoretic method, the enzyme activity in band two was higher
in gliomas and metastatic carcinomas than in band three, whereas no
marked differences were observed between bands two and three in neurinomas. Meningiomas and neuroblastomas revealed higher activities in band
three than in band two. In two glioblastomas, activity with acetyl-β-
methylthiocholine could not be demonstrated. Band three probably corresponds to acetylcholinesterase since the activity of this band was strongest
in the corpus striatum, although the substrate specificity of the thiocholin-
esterases is somewhat decreased compared to the more specific oxygen analogues. Inhibitors used for differentiating between acetyl- and butyrylcholinesterase (62C47 at 10^{-4} M concentration and Ro20683 at 10^{-6} M concentration) did not show selective effects because bands one and two were inhib-

TABLE XI

*Distribution of butyrylcholinesterase activity
in human brain tumours with BuTCH
as substrate on starch gel electrophoresis
(Figures represent percentage contribution of each band
to the total activity)*

Tumour No.	Band No.					
	+	3	2	1	0	—
Glioblastoma						
No. 174		18	82	—		
No. 411		—	100	—		
Glioblastoma						
No. 194		27	73	—		
No. 359		57	43	—		
Oligodendroglioma						
No. 150		35	65	—		
No. 350		67	33	—		
Astrocytoma						
No. 160		40	60			
Meningioma (end.)						
No. 193		30	70	—		
No. 432		29	71	—		
No. 197		27	73	—		
No. 440		44	56	—		
Meningioma (fibr.)						
No. 166		35	65	—		
Metastatic						
carcinoma		44	56	—		
No. 164		20	80	—		
No. 90						
Neurinoma		30	43	27		
No. 169		21	55	34		
No. 44						

ited completely and band three was unaffected by both inhibitors. Eserine at 10^{-4} M concentration inhibited all bands (see Figures 3.37, 3.47, 3.49).

To summarise the changes of cholinesterase activity in brain tumours, the high butyrylcholinesterase activity of gliomas is due to an activity increase in band two which is probably identical with serum cholinesterase. Isoenzymes with different electrophoretic mobilities were not observed. La Motta *et al.* (1961), transplanting glioblastoma multiforme in the anterior chamber of guinea pig eye, observed a decrease in the serum cholinesterase activity of the host. Human patients with nonhepatic carcinoma also exhibited low serum cholinesterase activities in the absence of low serum albumin. The authors proposed immunological suppression. According to our experiences serum cholinesterase activity was not lower in the serum or CSF of patients bearing glioblastoma or other brain tumours (Figures 3.38*a, b, c*; 3.50; 3.51).

TABLE XII

Distribution of acetylcholinesterase activity
in human brain tumours on starch gel electrophoresis
with MeTCH as substrate
(Figures represent percentage contribution of each band
to the total activity)

Tumour No.	Band No.					
	+	3	2	1	0	—
Glioblastoma						
No. 174		40	60	—		
No. 411		—	—	—		
No. 194		21	79	—		
No. 359		54	46	—		
No. 195		—	—	—		
Oligodendroglioma						
No. 150		42	58	—		
No. 350		16	84	—		
Astrocytoma						
No. 160		33	77	—		
Meningioma (end.)						
No. 193		84	16	—		
No. 432		50	50	—		
No. 197		51	49	—		
No. 440		73	27	—		
Meningioma (fibr.)						
No. 166		—	—	—		
Metastatic carcinoma						
No. 164		24	76	—		
No. 90		44	56	—		
Neurinoma						
No. 169		44	56	—		
No. 44		45	55	—		

According to Zacks (1958) several nonchromaffin paragangliomas exhibited cholinesterase activity with histochemical methods. Winkelmann (1960) also demonstrated nonspecific cholinesterase in neuroepithelial nevi.

The rôle of acetylcholinesterase in the nervous system is well known as the destruction of the chief neurotransmitter acetylcholine. In contrast much less is known about the function of butyrylcholinesterase. Cholinesterase in serum, liver and intestine has been attributed with a rôle in the cleavage of externally applied cholinesters or butyrylcholine formed during fat digestion (Clitherow et al. 1963, Jamieson 1963). According to Joo and Várkonyi (1969) butyrylcholinesterase is involved in the regulation of the blood brain barrier, presumably because of its rôle in transportation owing to its localisation in the pinocytotic vesicles of the cytoplasms of endothelial cells. No definite answer can be given in respect to the rôle of the increased butyrylcholinesterase activity of gliomas, since Cavanagh et al. (1954) did not observe a higher activity in the vascular elements of gliomas. However, increased cholinesterase activity was demonstrated by histochemical methods around blood vessels in some benign gliomas (Figure 3.39) (Wollemann 1970).

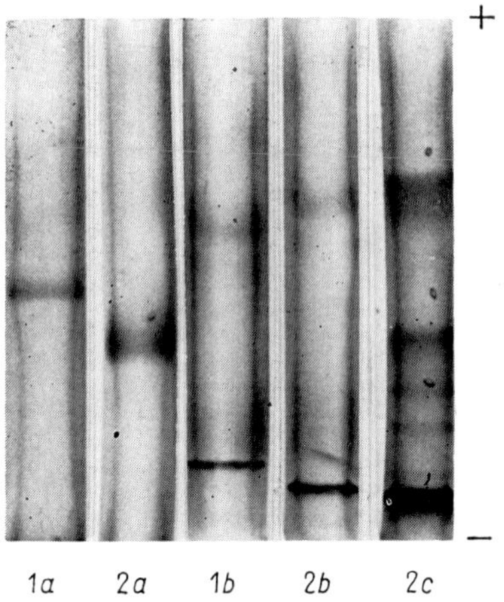

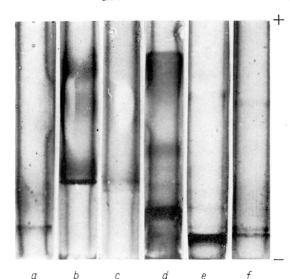

1a   2a   1b   2b   2c

Figure 3.38a. Cholinesterase and esterase patterns of glioblastoma No. 258 from tumour surrounding tissue (1), mitochondria (*a*) supernatant (*b*), serum (*c*) and tumour (2)

Aliesterase (B type esterase) hydrolyses aliphatic esters, preferentially tributyrin, but it is not strictly substrate specific since it also hydrolyses cholinesters and to a lesser degree aromatic esters. In contrast to cholinesterase it is not inhibited by 10^{-5} M eserine (which completely inhibits cholinesterase activity). Aliesterase is inhibited by alkylphosphates, as are cholinesterases. Aliesterase occurs in multiple forms in the blood plasma of lower vertebrates but it is absent in human, monkey, dog and pig plasma (Augustinsson 1961).

Pepler and Pearse (1957) differentiated between four types of aliesterases in the rat brain, using *o*-acetyl-5-bromoindoxylacetate as substrate and various concentrations of parathion and Mipafox as inhibitors. The main differ-

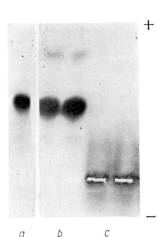

a   b   c   d   e   f

Figure 3.38b. Cholinesterase and esterase patterns of astrocytoma No. 282, mitochondrial fraction (*a*), supernatant (*b*), capsule (*c*), cyst (*d*), cyst of astrocytoma No. 132 (*e*) and neurinoma No. 138 (*f*)

a   b   c

Figure 3.38c. Cholinesterase and esterase patterns of serum (*a*), meningosarcoma No. 62 (*b*) and cystic fluid of spongioblastoma (*c*)

ences were encountered in the pH optimum, which varied between 2.1 and 8.0. According to Barron *et al.* (1963) human brain esterase isoenzymes revealed fifteen bands with α-naphthylacetate as substrate, five of them are classified as aliesterases. Bernsohn *et al.* (1966) showed that aliesterase was bound to the microsomal particles and was released by Triton X-100.

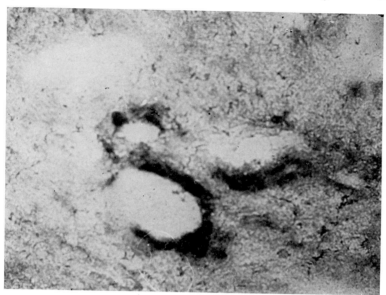

Figure 3.39. Cholinesterase activity of oligodendroglioma No. 150.
Increased activity in blood vessel walls. Magnification 100×

These data combined with the electron-microscopic and quantitative chemical analysis of the subcellular fractions of rat brain suggested that some bound nonspecific esterase may be present in the subsynaptic membranes. Histochemical methods revealed that aliesterase is localised in the cytoplasm of neurones and neuropil (Bernsohn *et al.* 1966).

Aliesterase activity was revealed after a short incubation almost exclusively in the astrocytes (Meyer-Ruge 1966) and was absent in neuroglia during embryonic development. Ecobichon and Kalow (1962) observed one aliesterase in human liver and Shaw and Koen (1963) reported a testosterone induced aliesterase in mouse kidney. According to the classification of Gomori (1952) aliesterases also include lipases, but brain revealed a very weak activity against long-chain esters of fatty acids with α and β-naphthols (Gomori 1955, Bernsohn *et al.* 1966).

Cavanagh *et al.*(1954) observed that tributyrin hydrolysis in brain tumours was increased in gliomas, similarly to pseudocholinesterase activity. The two enzyme activities were not completely parallel in the tumours and tributyrin cleavage was not inhibited by eserine, therefore a different enyzme activity was suggested for tributyrin hydrolysis. According to Barron *et al.* (1964) more organophosphate-sensitive esterase activity is present in the soluble fraction of neurofibroma than in normal brain. In astrocytoma the ratio of soluble/insoluble esterase is the same as in the normal brain, whereas in glioblastoma the pattern is totally different. However, according to Ecobichon (1966) and our experiences (1967) the majority of human brain esterases showed a nonspecific behaviour towards various esters and inhibitors.

The finding that liver aliesterase also hydrolyses amides, amino acid esters and long chain fatty acid esters suggests that esterase may play a part in protein and lipid metabolism (Myers *et al.* 1957, Hofstal 1960), although its rôle in brain function remains unclear.

Aromatic esterase (arylesterase or A-type esterase) is resistant to eserine and alkylphosphate, readily hydrolyses aromatic esters and does not attack aliphatic esters. Acetates are usually hydrolysed faster than propionates or butyrates. It is able to hydrolyse certain alkylphosphates and is inhibited by p-chloromercuribenzoate and activated by Ca^{2+} (Aldridge 1953, 1954, Augustinsson 1961). According to Bernsohn *et al.* (1966) aromatic esterase activity is localised in rat brain in particles (presumably lysosomes) of neurones and other cell types. According to the results obtained by the centrifugation of cell fractions, A-type esterase was localised in the supernatant, however, it was probably solubilised from the particles during isolation (Holt 1963, Bernsohn *et al.* 1966).

Aromatic esterase is present in the prealbumin and albumin fractions of human serum (Augustinsson 1959, Augustinsson and Brody 1962). Esterase occurring in multiple forms in red blood cells has been examined by starch gel electrophoresis (Tashian 1961, Shaw *et al.* 1962). Five basic types were distinguished, among which one (D esterase) was present also in an atypical form. The atypical enzyme is under genetic control and is a variant form of erythrocyte carbonic anhydrase.

Arylesterase was studied by electrophoretic techniques in human and rat brain by several authors. Using different naphthol esters as substrate, 10–15–18 bands appeared (Barron *et al.* 1961, 1963, Eränkö *et al.* 1962, Ecobichon 1966). Only slight quantitative differences were observed in the various regions. The number of human esterase isoenzymes was considerably greater than those observed in rat, rabbit, cat or guinea pig. Difficulties were encountered in the classification using organophosphate inhibitors since parathion and TEPP-sensitive bands were resistant to DFP and sensitive to p-chloromercuribenzoate inhibition (Barron *et al.* 1963), however, they fit in with the fluoride, DFP insensitive 'general' esterase type of Gomori (1955). According to Gerhardt *et al.* (1963) four anodic and 6–7 cathodic bands showing esterase activity were found in normal human brain by agar gel electrophoresis. By using selective inhibitors, the slower prealbumin and two β-globulin bands were identified as cholinesterase, the five cathodic bands were classified as nonspecific esterases, and an intensely stained slow α-globulin band showed aromatic esterase activity. Quantitative differences were also observed among the different brain regions.

Our own results (Wollemann *et al.* 1965, Wollemann 1967, 1970) revealed ten isoenzymes on starch gel electrophoresis using α-naphthylacetate as

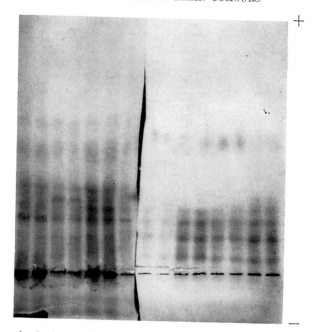

1 1 2 2 3 3 4 4 4 3 3 2 2 1 1

Figure 3.40. Protein (*a*) and esterase (*b*) patterns of supernatants of various areas of normal human brain after starch gel electrophoresis: nucleus caudatus and putamen (1), cerebellar cortex (2), cortical grey matter (3) and subcortical white matter (4)

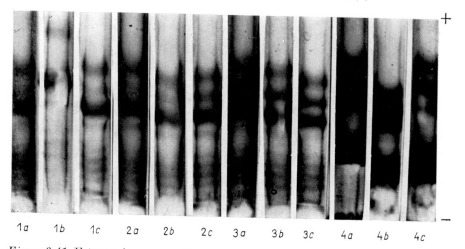

1a 1b 1c 2a 2b 2c 3a 3b 3c 4a 4b 4c

Figure 3.41. Esterase isoenzymes from twenty-six weeks old human embryonic brain: cortical grey matter (1), subcortical white matter (2), thalamus (3), hypothalamus (4), control (*a*), treated with 10^{-5} M eserine (*b*), and with 10^{-5} M DFP (*c*)

substrate. Two isoenzymes moved towards the cathode and eight towards the anode (Figures 3.40, 3.50). Three anodic bands were identified as cholinesterases on the basis of eserine sensitivity and substrate specificity. All bands were sensitive to 10^{-5} M parathion. The esterase pattern changed during development. According to several authors using starch gel electrophoresis (Lagnado and Hardy 1965) and polyacrylamide disc electrophoresis (Wollemann et al. 1971a), with α-naphthylacetate as substrate, slow moving bands were absent in 4–8 months old human foetuses (Figure 3.41). Bernsohn et al. (1965) did not demonstrate arylesterase activity in white matter of the cerebrum with α-naphthylpropionate until 4–5 months.

Changes in the esterase pattern of rat brain and serum following cranial X-ray irradiation were also encountered (Masurovsky and Noback 1963).

Quantitative measurements in the supernatant fraction of normal brain and brain tumour homogenates in the presence of α-naphthylacetate as substrate and 10^{-4} M eserine as inhibitor of cholinesterase activity revealed the highest rates of hydrolysis in meningiomas and neurinomas (Wollemann 1970) (see Tables XIII, XIV), whereas gliomas revealed lower eserine resistant esterase and higher cholinesterase values.

TABLE XIII

The rates of hydrolysis of various substrates by concentrated supernatants from different areas of normal human brain
(Results are expressed as μmol substrate hydrolysed/mg protein/hour)

Area	α-NA (2.4×10⁻² M)		ACH (3×10⁻³ M)	BuCH (2×10⁻² M)	MeCH (7×10⁻³ M)
Substrate / Inhibitor	—	Eserine (10⁻⁴ M)	—	—	—
Caudate nucleus and putamen	3.6 3.4	0.2 0.1	3.4 3.1	0.4 0.3	1.6 1.2
Cerebellar cortex	2.1 1.6	0.8 0.7	0.9 0.6 0.5	0.3 0.3 0.3	0.5 0.4
Cerebral cortex	1.5 1.0	0.7 0.6	0.5 0.4 0.4	0.2 0.1 0.1	0.2 0.2
Subcortical white matter	1.1 0.7	0.5 0.3	0.2 0.2 0.2	0.3 0.3 0.2	0.1 0.1

The localisation of the nonspecific aromatic esterase in brain tumours was, according to Müller and Nasu (1962), similar to that of acid phosphatase. The esterase activity in neurinomas was scattered throughout the whole cell plasma but there was no difference between the Antoni A and B areas. The histochemical distribution of esterase in glioblastomas (Figure 3.42) and one malignant astrocytoma (Figure 3.43) suggests that a great part of the activity is contributed by tumour astrocytes, which show a relatively high degree of differentiation. Intense esterase activity was present in the reactive microglia around the necrotic areas of malignant gliomas and meta-static carcinomas (Figure 3.44). The proliferating blood vessels of glioblas-tomas (Figure 3.47) showed low enzyme activities, in oligodendrogliomas the activity was also completely absent in the vascular stroma, whereas in benign astrocytoma the blood vessels were well outlined (Wollemann *et al.* 1965, Wollemann 1970) (Figure 3.45). The esterase activity of meningiomas showed marmorate patterns and zones of intense activity at the periphery of the lobules alternating with central areas of low activity (Figure 3.46).

The aromatic esterase activity increases generally during cell cultivation similarly to other lysosomal enzymes during an increase of catabolic activity (Matakas 1969).

TABLE XIV

The rates of hydrolysis of various substrates by concentrated supernatants from the human brain tumours in the presence and absence of inhibitors (Results are expressed as µmol of substrate hydrolysed/mg protein)

Tumour / Substrate / Inhibitor	α-NA (2.4×10^{-2} M)		ACH (3×10^{-3} M)		BuCH (2×10^{-2} M)		MeCH (7×10^{-3} M)
	—	Eserine (10^{-4} M)	—	62C47 (10^{-4} M)	—	RO2-0683 (10^{-4} M)	—
Glioblastoma							
No. 194			1.0		2.7		
No. 174			1.1	0.1	2.1	0.0*	
No. 411			0.8		2.5		0.0
No. 359	3.5	0.5	1.5		2.4		0.3
No. 195	3.2	0.3	1.0		2.5		0.1
No. 949	3.1	0.3	1.3		2.6		
Oligodendroglioma							
No. 150			1.1	0.2	2.9	1.1	
No. 350			1.3		2.1		
Astrocytoma							
No. 160			0.5	0.2	1.4	0.5	
Meningioma (end.)							
No. 193			0.1		0.8		
No. 432			0.2		0.6		
No. 440	1.5	0.8	0.4	0.1	0.4		0.1
No. 197	2.3	1.1	0.5		0.5		0.1
No. 348	1.4	0.6					
Meningioma (fibr.)							
No. 166			0.1		0.1		0.02
Metastatic carcinoma							
No. 164			0.3		0.2		0.2
No. 90	1.9	0.2	1.1	0.2	1.1	0.3	0.5
No. 167	1.3	0.3					
Neurinoma							
No. 169	1.5	0.6	0.5		0.8		0.4
No. 47			0.2		0.2		

* RO2-0683 (5×10^{-5} M)

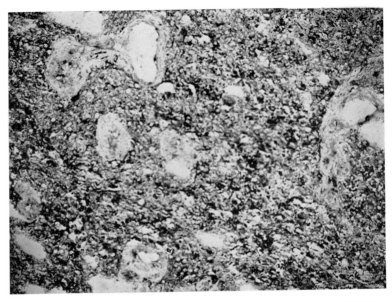

Figure 3.42. Esterase activity of glioblastoma multiforme No. 195. Moderate enzyme activity with some variation in the intensity of staining in individual tumour cells. The blood vessel walls show little or no enzyme activity. Magnification 120 ×

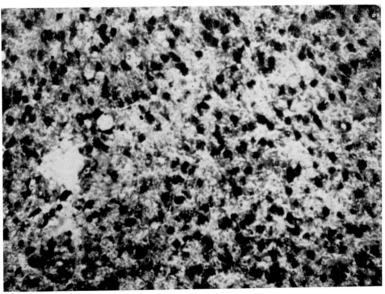

Figure 3.43. Esterase activity of gemistocytic astrocytoma No. 160. Intense activity is seen in astrocytic tumour cells. Magnification 160 ×

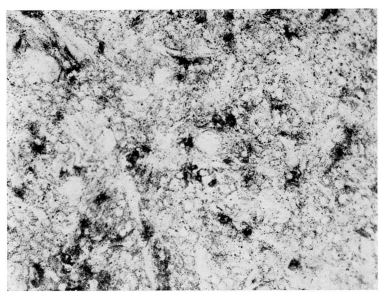

Figure 3.44. Esterase activity of metastatic carcinoma No. 167 infiltrating the dura. Intense activity in pleomorphic microglial cells infiltrating the dura in response to its invasion by secondary carcinoma. The outline of the unstained tumour nuclei can be identified. Magnification 100 ×

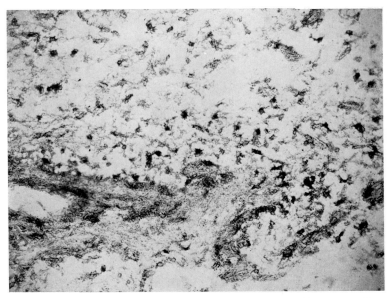

Figure 3.45. Esterase activity of cerebellar astrocytoma No. 126. Considerable reaction in individual stellate astrocytic tumour cells, mostly around the blood vessels. Magnification 140 ×

10*

A changed esterase isoenzyme pattern in brain tumours was demonstrated by different gel electrophoretic methods. Gerhardt *et al.* (1963) observed in some glioblastomas double bands and a changed electrophoretic mobility in the slower moving prealbumin fraction. Serum cholinesterase bands were present in gliomas. Cathodal esterase activities were low in malignant tumours and high in meningiomas as revealed by agar gel electrophoresis.

Bands of relatively low intensity were demonstrated when staining for esterase activity in the prealbumin and albumin fractions of glioblastomas and strong activities were present in the bands which originated from serum cholinesterase. In benign gliomas and meningiomas 10–13 bands of esterase activity, usually 2–3 with prealbumin mobility, were encountered. Metastatic carcinomas showed similar patterns to glioblastomas. One malignant fibroblastic meningioma and neurinomas also showed esterase patterns similar to glioblastomas (see Table XV and Figures 3.47–3.51) (Wollemann *et al.* 1965, Wollemann 1967, 1970). All esterase bands in the tumours were inhibited by parathion.

There is no correlation between the esterase pattern of malignant tumours and the pattern of embryonic brain tissue, since in the foetal brain the low mobility bands (presumably cholinesterase) are absent and high mobility bands are dominant. Another example of the dissimilarity of brain tumours and embryonic tissue is the creatine phosphotransferase isoenzyme pattern (see page 113).

Gomori (1955) studied over one hundred various human tumours by histochemical esterase techniques. He established, by using different inhib-

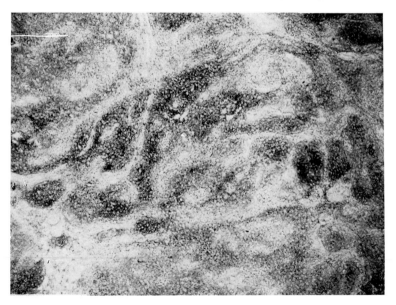

Figure 3.46. Esterase activity of endotheliomatous meningioma. Note the pattern of alternating zones of high and low enzyme activity. The connective tissue stroma shows no enzyme activity. Magnification 78×

TABLE XV

Distribution of aromatic esterase activity in human brain tumours on starch gel electrophoresis
(Figures represent percentage contribution of each band to the total activity)

Tumour No.	+	11	10	9	8	7	6	5	4	3	2	1	0	1	2	−
Glioblastoma																
No. 174		—	—	—	—	—	2	6	40	24	11	7		5	4	
No. 411		—	—	—	—	2	3	7	48	12	13	7		7	1	
No. 194		—	—	—	1	1	7	11	21	11	20	27		—	—	
No. 359		—	—	—	5	6	7	7	28	16	11	10		10	1	
No. 195		—	—	—	—	—	—	—	37	20	19	25		—	—	
Oligodendroglioma																
No. 150		—	3	23	8	11	7	9	11	11	6	7		4	1	
No. 350		—	—	24	20	1	2	6	17	5	7	18		—	—	
No. 257		—	—	26	11	1	1	4	22	8	6	9		6	7	
Astrocytoma																
No. 160		9	—	10	4	3	7	7	35	4	5	4		13	9	
No. 126		—	11	15	8	3	12	4	13	11	3	3		4	2	
Meningioma (end.)																
No. 193		11	30	16	1	2	1	4	14	4	10	2		3	2	
No. 432		—	2	2	1	1	2	3	18	11	11	33		12	3	
No. 440		—	—	2	9	5	5	4	14	11	15	13		13	14	
Meningioma (fibr.)																
No. 166		—	—	4	4	2	3	4	27	10	11	10		13	11	
Metastatic carcinoma																
No. 164		—	1	1	—	—	2	5	41	13	21	7		7	2	
No. 90		—	—	—	5	9	11	6	23	15	10	21		—	—	
Neurinoma																
No. 169		—	—	5	16	2	2	4	60	2	5	3		—	—	
No. 47		—	—	9	4	6	6	9	26	12	9	10		3	4	

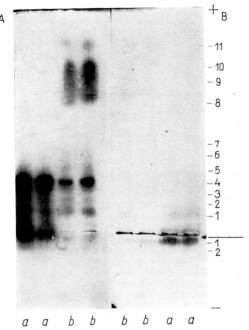

Figure 3.47. Esterase patterns of supernatants of brain tumours after starch gel electrophoresis: glioblastoma multiforme No. 411 (*a*), meningioma endothel. No. 193 (*b*); B = esterase activity inhibited with 10^{-4} M eserine

itors and substrates, that the esterase type was identical with the parent tissue in hepatomas and tumours of pancreatic, thyroid, prostatic and bronchial origin. Brain tumours are, however, different in this respect, as seen above.

Studies of normal human cells and tumour cells grown *in vitro* have shown seventeen nonspecific carboxylic esterases with eight or more subgroups. The patterns did not change during cell culture (Komma 1963).

Esterase isoenzyme patterns in Rous sarcoma virus induced tumours in the rat showed a pattern different from normal tissue. When the tumour was explanted in tissue culture the isoenzyme pattern changed again (Levan *et al.* 1971).

Only indirect conclusions can be drawn on the function of arylesterases in the brain. The lysosomal localisation and the appearance of esterase during the critical period in brain maturation suggest a catabolic or transport action of the enzyme, since lysosomes give rise to pinocytotic and autophagic vacuoles. Accord- ing to De Duve (1959, 1963) and Essner (1960) they play an important part in phagocytosis, digestion, transcellular transport, necrosis and autolysis. These functions are also involved during the growth and necrosis of tumours.

Cathepsin-like C esterase also attacks carboxylic esters, but it differs from A and B-type esterase in that it is activated by low concentrations of *p*-chlormercuribenzoate. It is not inhibited by eserine and alkylphosphates in contrast to B esterase, but is similar to A esterase in that it does not hydrolyse alkylphosphates (Bergmann *et al.* 1957, Bergmann and Rimon 1958).

C esterase was localised in the lysosomes in brain by several authors. Torack and Barnett (1962) established its presence from the hydrolysis of thiolacetic acid and Beaufay *et al.* (1957) and Koenig *et al.* (1964) demonstrated C esterase activity by cell fractionation methods. Bernsohn *et al.* (1966) concluded that it occurs in both soluble and bound forms in brain. According to the same authors (Barron *et al.* 1963) C-type esterase activity is revealed by starch gel electrophoresis of normal brain tissue in esterase band eleven migrating towards the anode. This band was activated by p-chloromercuribenzoate and was resistant to organophosphate inhibition, but the histochemical localisation with p-chloromercuribenzoate activation did not show discernible effects. Hence the type of lysosomal esterase is still open to histochemical investigations.

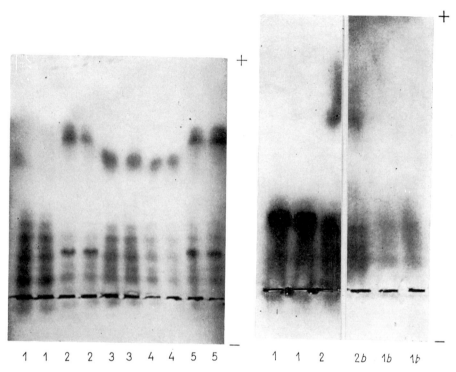

Figure 3.48. Esterase patterns of super-natants of normal brain and brain tu-mours after starch gel electrophoresis: caudate nucleus and putamen (1), menin-gioma endothel. No. 193 (2), cortical grey matter (3), subcorticalwhitematter (4) and meningioma endothel. No. 193 (5)

Figure 3.49. Esterase patterns of su-pernatants of brain tumours after starch gel electrophoresis: glioblas-toma multiforme No. 174 (1), oligo-dendroglioma No. 350 (2), esterase activity inhibited with 10^{-4} M eser-ine (b)

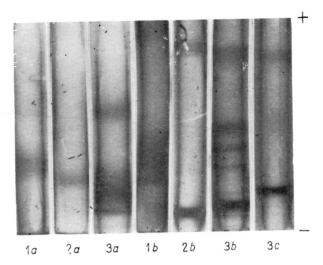

1a   2a   3a   1b   2b   3b   3c

Figure 3.50. Esterase and cholinesterase patterns
from different cell fractions of astrocytoma No. 33,
tumour surrounding tissue (*a*), tumour (*b*) and serum
(*c*); nuclear (1), mitochondrial (2) and supernatant (3)
cell fractions

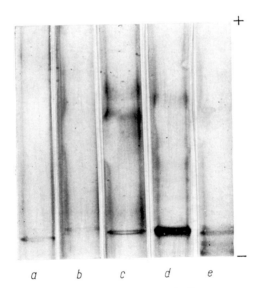

a   b   c   d   e

Figure 3.51. Esterase and cholinesterase
patterns from different cell fractions
and CFS of medulloblastoma No. 279,
nuclear (*a*), mitochondrial (*b*) and supernatant (*c*) cell fractions, CSF (*d*) and
CSF of encephalitis No. 278 (*e*)

4. Glycosidases

Glycosidases are hydrolases which split glycosidic linkages. The glycosidic linkage consists of a bond between the aldehyde group of a sugar (glycone moiety) and a hydroxyl group of another compound (aglycone moiety). In brain tumours, β-glucuronidase and β-galactosidase have been investigated.

β-glucuronidase catalyses the hydrolysis of conjugated aromatic β-D-glucuronides. Among mammalian tissues, liver, kidney, spleen and epididymis exhibited highest activities. De Duve *et al.* (1955), using cel fractionation methods, found that the enzyme was localised in the lysosomes. The pH optimum of β-glucuronidase is between 4.5 and 5.2 (Fishman 1950). β-glucuronidase in brain is also localised in the lysosomal particles. It is present both in the neurones and glial cells according to Fishman and Hayashi (1962). Pearse (1961) established strong β-glucuronidase activity in the choroid plexus and in the Purkinje cells. Waltimo and Talanti (1965) demonstrated high activities in the pineal gland of rat brain and in the hypothalamic magnocellular neurosecretory nuclei. From these data it may be suggested that β-glucuronidase activity is localised in the parts of the brain with a secretory function with the exception of the Purkinje cells. The β-glucuronidase activity is selectively inhibited by saccharo-γ-lactones (Levvy 1952).

Lehrer (1962) reported 6–30 times increased β-glucuronidase activities; the highest levels were demonstrated in two of the most malignant gliomas. According to Lehrer (1962) an increase in β-glucuronidase activity is associated with active growth in glial cells. He concluded therefore that the increase in enzyme activity in gliomas may be correlated with the growth rate in glial cells. Allen (1961, 1962) investigated thirty-six brain tumours and reported similarly increased levels of β-glucuronidase activity but there was no consistent relationship with regard to histochemical malignancy. In the glioma group, however, the more anaplastic tumours tend to have higher activities. The increase of β-glucuronidase activity in the different types of tumours, such as medulloblastoma, neuroblastoma, neurinoma, meningioma and metastatic carcinoma, rather suggests that the origin of the increased activity might be the enhancement of lysosomal acid hydrolase activities.

A high β-glucuronidase activity was also encountered in some other neoplasms. Fishman (1950, 1955) and Fishman and Mitchell (1959) showed that several primary human neoplasms from skin, lung, breast, gastrointestinal tract, uterine cervix and brain showed high β-glucuronidase activities compared with adjacent normal brain tissue. The stromal activity of cancer tissue was variable. Monis *et al.* (1960) confirmed these results and they also observed that malignant epithelial tumours generally exhibited an intense activity in contrast to mesenchymal tumours which showed little or no activity. These observations, however, do not correlate with mesenchymal brain tumour activities, because neurinomas and meningiomas also exhibited high β-glucuronidase activities.

β-galactosidase, the second enzyme among glycosidases investigated in brain tumours, hydrolyses β-D-galactosides. β-galactosidase activity occurs in mammalian intestine, liver, skeletal muscle, stomach, kidney, pancreas, heart and brain. β-galactosidase with a pH optimum around three has been found in the lysosomes (Maio and Rickenberg 1960, Sellinger *et al.* 1960). In the cat small intestinal mucosa it has been reported to consist of two different forms: a neutral and an acid enzyme. The molecular weight of the neutral enzyme is 3–5 times higher than that of the acid enzyme (Kraml *et al.* 1970). Human small intestine contains three forms of β-galactosidase, a monomer, a dimer and an octa- or polymer (Asp 1971). β-galactosidase is inhibited by galactoselactone and p-chloromercuribenzoate. Beef liver contained two components of β-galactosidase according to Chytil (1965), whereas four fractions were present in rat liver lysosomes.

β-galactosidase was the first enzyme shown to be inducible in the presence of three genes and substrate in *E. coli* (Jacob and Monod 1961). In the non-induced strains of *E. coli* only one form of β-galactosidase was revealed by disc gel electrophoresis (Appel *et al.* 1965). After induction with isopropyl-β-D-thiogalactoside, seven forms of the enzyme were resolved by acrylamide gel electrophoresis. The multiple forms differed from each other in molecular weight.

β-galactosidase was also investigated in cell cultures of brain tumours where the activity was found to be increased, as with other hydrolases, irrespective of the type of tumour (Matakas 1969).

β-galactosidase is involved in several genetic diseases where the loss of lysosomal hydrolases is a characteristic feature. The lack of hydrolases results in a simultaneous accumulation of mucopolysaccharides and complex lipids (Van Hoof 1970).

*

In summarising the results of hydrolases, the discovery of lysosomes by cell fractionating and histochemical methods was very important in the pathogenesis of brain tumours. The rôle of the hydrolases in the lysosomes is the enzymic digestion of the pathologically altered, degenerated or necrotic cells, according to their proteolytic, lipolytic, phosphorolytic or glycosidic function. These properties could be useful to some extent for diagnostic and therapeutic purposes, but the increase in hydrolase activity does not provide suitable means for classifying the type of tumour.

Changes of Hydrolase Activity in Brain Tumours

Enzyme activity	Type of brain tumour													
	GL	MT	GB	AC	OG	EM	SB	MB	NN	MG	MC	SC	NB	EI
Alkaline phosphatase	+[5] +[6]				−[13]	+[18]			+[19]	+[1] +[15-17]		−[19] −[7]		−[19]
Acid phosphatase	+[2] +[3] +[14]								−[19] +[2]	+[2]				
Esterase	+[2] +[3] +[14] +[7]								−[19] +[7]	+[2] +[7]				
Acetylcholinesterase	−[10] −[11] −[12]		−[12]	−[12]			−[10] −[11] −[12]			−[10] −[11] −[12]	−[10] −[11] −[12]		+[22]	
Butyrylcholinesterase	+[9-12]		+[9-11]	+[9-11]										
β-Glucuronidase	+[4] +[8] +[20]	+[4]						+[4] +[21]	+[4] +[21]	+[4] +[21]	+[4] +[21]		+[4] +[21]	
β-Galactosidase	+[7]													

+ = increase. − = decrease.

[1] Friede (1956), [2] Wollemann et al. (1965), [3] Wollemann (1970), [4] Lehrer (1962), [5] Udvarhelyi et al. (1962) [6] Viale and Andreussi (1965), [7] Matakas (1969), [8] Sano et al. (1966), [9] Youngstrom et al. (1941), [10] Cavanagh et al. (1954), [11] Bülbring et al. (1953), [12] Wollemann and Zoltán (1962), [13] Kreuzberg and Gullotta (1967), [14] Sutton and Becker (1969), [15] Landow et al. (1942), [16] Büttger et al. (1957), [17] Feigen and Wolf (1958), [18] Kirsch (1963), [19] Müller and Nasu (1960), [20] Allen (1961), [21] Lehrer (1962a), [22] Kates et al. (1971).

4. SUMMARY, CONCLUSIONS AND FUTURE TRENDS

Considering the most important results revealed in brain tumour bio-chemistry and comparing them with results obtained in general oncology, the following conclusions may be drawn.

Among pathochemical changes in the polysaccharides, high glycogen levels in some gliomas, with the exception of oligodendrogliomas, reflect an increase of glycogen storage as compared to normal brain. Similar results were obtained in other malignant tumours. The enzymic activities of gly-cogen synthesis and breakdown (glycogen synthetase and phosphorylase) were both shown to be reduced. Increased anaerobic glycolysis in malignant tumours is supplied by the direct phosphorylation of glucose at the hexo-kinase level. Thus the increased glycogen content in brain tumours plays only a secondary rôle as an energy store in glucose metabolism.

An interesting new approach to molecular tumour genesis is given by Weber and Lea (1965). Differentiating between slow, medium and rapidly growing hepatomas, they reported that a decrease of gluconeogenesis and an increase of glycolysis and glucose oxidation was parallel with an increase in growth rate. Together with the decrease of gluconeogenic enzymes, their induction with steroids also ceased. A similar pattern can be outlined for the slow, medium and rapidly growing gliomas.

An increase in certain acid mucopolysaccharides partly bound to protein is also characteristic of brain tumour glial cells, and changes in glycolipids possessing antigenic properties also reflect differences used in the immune-diagnosis of brain tumours. The changes in lipid content are characterised by low phospholipid values, attributed mainly to the phosphoethanolamine containing cephalin fraction. In contrast, the ^{32}P uptake was increased in the phospholipid fraction, usually in the cell rich brain tumours. The relative increase in cell lipids, esterified cholesterol and fatty acids in the cell mem-brane indicates changes in cell permeability. The increased cholesterol metabolism is parallel to the malignancy in the glioma group and similar to the cholesterol metabolism of embryonic brain. The fatty acids of brain tumours were different from normal brain, as well as from blood plasma fatty acids.

Changes in brain tumour protein fractions have been reported, but these were only quantitative or not consistent. Variations in the CSF protein fractions as revealed by the different gel electrophoretic methods were not characteristic for brain tumours alone, although the capacity of brain tissue to produce different immunoglobulins in various diseases of the CNS —among others brain tumours—is noteworthy. Comparison of protein fractions from serum, CSF, cystic fluid and tumours might be useful for investigating the origin of the increased protein fraction in the CSF. An increased uptake of radioiodinated serum albumin into brain tumours, owing to the increased permeability and pinocytosis, is used in the diagnosis of brain tumours.

High levels of DNA in malignant brain tumours were reported, especially in the large cell type of glioblastoma and medulloblastoma as well as in experimentally induced brain gliomas. Methylated bases occurred more frequently in the tumours, as well as in embryonic brain, in comparison to normal adult brain.

The oxidative and glycolytic metabolism of brain tumours is characterised by a low respiratory and high glycolytic activity, which corresponds to the malignancy. Respiratory enzymic activity is relatively high in oligodendrogliomas and benign astrocytomas, with a high rate of reactive and gemistocytic astrocytes. The number and form of mitochondria and the respiratory enzymic equipment does not keep level with the increased energy requirement of the fast growing tumours and therefore glycolysis is increased. In addition, the structure of some glycolytic enzymes is altered showing similarities with the embryonic enzyme structure. Examples of this kind of charged protein structure are lactic dehydrogenase and aldolase. Differences in enzymic structure occur also in enzymes which are represented by various forms in the cytoplasm and the cell particles. A typical example is the change in the soluble and mitochondrial malate dehydrogenase isoenzymes in brain tumours. A return to the embryonic molecular pattern of some brain tumour enzymes is, however, not a general rule for changed brain tumour isoenzyme patterns, but it reflects rather an adaptation to the metabolic requirements of tumour growth. An example of this concept is the creatine phosphotransferase isoenzyme. Creatine phosphotransferase isoenzymes in the brain are not changed during development, embryo and adult brains showing the same pattern. However, the isoenzyme pattern of malignant brain tumours is changed, because isoenzymes of the muscle type appear. Similar alterations occur in the esterase isoenzyme pattern.

It is not difficult to predict that, owing to the investigations on the rôle of isoenzymes as genetic markers, the demonstration of isoenzymes will occupy an important place in future brain tumour research. Molecular pathology is now able to use the results of the changed isoenzyme patterns for both diagnostic and aetiological conclusions.

A common feature of brain tumours is the loss of specific nervous function, thus neurotransmitter metabolism is absent with the exception of special transmitter producing neoplasms, for instance neuroblastoma and phaeochromocytoma, which are primary tumours of the peripheral nervous system. In gliomas and tumours of mesenchymal origin, enzymes of acetylcholine, GABA, serotonin or catecholamine metabolism are decreased or absent.

The general conclusions of Weber and Lea (1965) obtained on hepatomas with respect to the different growth rate—concerning protein and nucleic acid metabolism—seem to be also valid in the glioma tumour group. The synthetic reactions of protein and nucleic acid metabolism are increased and the catabolic reactions decreased in the faster growing tumours. An additional factor in brain tumours is the increased activity of lysosomal hydrolytic enzymes, which are present not only in the tumour cells, but also in the microglia, macrophages and reactive cells.

The most fascinating problem of tumour genesis for the biochemist is its molecular mechanism. Whatever the nature of the tumour inducing agent, its point of attack is ultimately the changed cell replicating mechanism and is therefore on the level of DNA and RNA synthesis. This presumption is supported by several results reported in the last years, such as the occurrence of special transfer and ribosomal RNAs observed in brain tumours and the increased incorporation of nucleotides in DNA. Earlier investigations pointed to an increased ^{32}P uptake into nucleic acids and an increased ribose synthesis in brain tumours. Yet the main evidence will come perhaps from the tumour producing virus investigations; virus RNA dependent DNA polymerase is one of the proven tumour producing mechanisms (Temin and Mizutani 1970, Baltimore 1970, Fujinaga et al. 1970, Gallo et al. 1970). Until the final mechanism of the development of brain tumours is explained, the changes in the two gene dependent isoenzyme synthesis will be expected to throw more light on this mechanism.

The histologically different types of brain tumours are also reflected in different metabolic patterns. The metabolic changes are more sensitive than the morphological alterations, because alterations occur first at the molecular level, and their histological equivalent will be apparent only at a later period, when rough differences are manifested. Therefore the search for demonstrating tumour specific substances by different immunological, electrophoretic, isotopic, electron-microscopic and other biochemical methods will be widely applied in brain tumour diagnosis in the future. Chemotherapy will be used not only in hopeless cases, or as a complementary treatment to surgery, but perhaps in the not too distant future as the most effective therapy against tumours. The establishment of the molecular mechanism of normal brain functions, the tissue culture of brain tumour cells, the influence of the blood-brain permeability will also help these efforts.

It is now much easier to predict these things than it was eighty-seven years ago for Thudichum, who wrote in his treatise on the chemical constitution of brain:

> I believe that the great disease of the brain and spine, . . .will all be shown to be connected with specific chemical changes in neuroplasm, the products of which cannot be more complicated than the chemolytic products of the ducts; they need, however, not be identical with chemolytic products but may be new morbid products . . . The knowledge of the composition and properties of neuroplasm and of its constituents will also aid us in devising modes of radical treatment in cases in which at present only tentative symptomatic measures are taken.

Probably a hundred years after Thudichum's predictions many of his forecasts will be accomplished, among them the solution of the brain tumour problem. One can be at least as optimistic as Shelley and ask, 'If Winter comes, can Spring be far behind?'

ABBREVIATIONS

A   = adrenaline
ACH   = acetylcholine
AC   = astrocytoma
ACHE   = acetylcholinesterase
ADP   = adenosine diphosphate
AKGA   = α-ketoglutaric acid
AMP   = 5′-adenosine monophosphate
ATCH   = acetylthiocholine
ATP   = adenosine triphosphate
BCHE   = butyrylcholinesterase
BOL   = bromo-lisergic acid
BuCH   = butyrylcholine
BuTCH   = butyrylthiocholine
BT   = benign tumour
CAMP   = cyclic 3′5′-adenosine monophosphate
CHE   = cholinesterase
CNS   = central nervous system
CoA   = coenzyme A
CP   = craniopharyngeoma
CrPK   = creatine phosphokinase
CSF   = cerebrospinal fluid
Cyt   = cytochrome
DCI   = dichloroisoproterenol
DFP   = diisopropylfluorophosphate
DES   = diethylstilboestrol
DNA   = deoxyribonucleic acid
DOPA   = dihydroxyphenylalanine
EDTA   = ethylenediamine tetraacetate
EI   = experimentally induced tumour
EM   = ependymoma
end   = endotheliomatous
ENZ   = enzyme
FAD   = flavine adenine dinucleotide
fibr.   = fibromatous
FMN   = flavine mononucleotide
FMNH$_2$ = reduced flavine mononucleotide
GABA   = γ-aminobutyric acid
GABA-T   = γ-aminobutyric acid transferase
GAD   = glutamic acid decarboxylase
GB   = glioblastoma multiforme
GDH   = glutamic acid dehydrogenase
GDP   = guanosine diphosphate
GL   = glioma
GOT   = glutamic-oxalacetic acid transferase
G-6-PDH   = glucose-6-phosphate dehydrogenase
GTP   = guanosine triphosphate
HG   = haptoglobin

HMP	=	hexose monophosphate
ICDH	=	isocitric acid dehydrogenase
LDH	=	lactic acid dehydrogenase
LP	=	lipoprotein
LSD	=	lysergic acid diethylamine
MAO	=	monoaminooxidase
MB	=	medulloblastoma
MC	=	metastatic carcinoma
MDH	=	malic acid dehydrogenase
MeCH	=	acetyl-β-methylcholine
MeTCH	=	acetyl-β-methylthiocholine
MG	=	meningioma
NMT	=	α-methyl-m-tyrosine
MPS	=	mucopolysaccharide
MT	=	malignant tumour
NA	=	noradrenaline
α-NA	=	α-naphthylacetate
NAD	=	nicotinamide adenine dinucleotide
NADH	=	reduced nicotinamide adenine dinucleotide
NADP	=	nicotinamide dinucleotide phosphate
NADPH	=	reduced nicotinamide dinucleotide phosphate
NB	=	neuroblastoma
NN	=	neurinoma
OD	=	optical density
OG	=	oligodendroglioma
4-OHB	=	4-hydroxybutyric acid
OMPA	=	octamethylpyrophosphate tetramide
PAS	=	periodic acid schiff reaction
PP	=	pyridoxal phosphate
RNA	=	ribonucleic acid
RQ	=	respiratory quotient
SB	=	spongioblastoma
SC	=	sarcoma
SDH	=	succinate dehydrogenase
SSA	=	succinic semialdehyde
TEPP	=	tetraethylpyrophosphate
TM 10	=	choline-2,6-xylyl ether
TS	=	tumour surrounding tissue
VMA	=	3-methoxy-4-hydroxymandelic acid

REFERENCES

Abood, L. G., Gerard, R. W., Banks, J. and Tschirgi, R. D. *Amer. J. Physiol.*, **168** 728, 1952.

Abood, l. G. and Romanchek, L. *Biochem. J.*, **60**, 233, 1955.

Abood, L. G. and Abul Haj, S. K. *J. Neurochem.*, **1**, 119, 1956.

Abood, L. G. and Alexander, L. *J. biol. Chem.*, **227**, 717, 1957.

Ács, G., Ostrowski, W. and Straub, F. B. *Acta physiol. Acad. Sci. hung.*, **6**, 261, 1954.

Ács, G., Garzo, T., Grosz, G., Molnár, J., Stephaneck, O. and Straub, F. B. *Acta physiol. Acad. Sci. hung.*, **8**, 269, 1955.

Ács, G., Neidle, A. and Waelsch, H. *Biochim. biophys. Acta (Amst.)*, **50**, 403, 1961.

Ács, G. and Reich, E.: *Antibiotics Mechanism of Action* (Eds D. Gottlieb and P. D. Shaw, Springer Verlag, New York, 1967, p. 494.

Adams, C. W. M. and Davison, A. N. *J. Neurochem.* **4**, 282, 1959.

Adams, C. W. M. and Davison, A. N. *J. Neurochem.*, **5**, 293, 1960.

Adelstein, S. J. and Vallee, B. L. *J. biol. Chem.*, **233**, 589, 1958.

Adler, E., Euler, H. V., Günther, G. and Plass, M. *Biochem. J.* **33**, 1028, 1939.

Aeberhard, E. and Menkes, J. H. *J. biol. Chem.*, **243**, 3834, 1968.

Agostini, A., Vergani, C. and Villa, L. *Nature (Lond.)*, **209**, 1024, 1966.

Agranoff, B. W. Cytidine Nucleotides. In *The Neurochemistry of Nucleotides and Amino Acids.* (Eds R. O. Brady and B. Tower), John Wiley, New York, 1960, p. 38.

Aisenberg, A. C. *The Glycolysis and Respiration of Tumors,* Academic Press, New York, 1961.

Akerfeldt, S. *Science, N.Y.*, **125**, 117, 1957.

Aldridge, W. N. *Biochem. J.*, **53**, 110, 1953.

Aldridge, W. N. *Biochem. J.*, **57**, 693, 1954.

Aldridge, W. N. and Johnson, M. K. *Biochem. J.*, **73**, 270, 1959.

Allen, N. *J. Neurochem.*, **2**, 37, 1957.

Allen, N. *Neurology (Minneap.)*, **11**, 578, 1961.

Allen, N. *IV. International Congress of Neuropathology, Proceedings*, Vol. I. (Ed. H. Jacob), G. Thieme Verlag, Stuttgart, 1962, p. 104.

Alles, G. A. and Hawes, R. C. *J. biol. Chem.*, **133**, 375, 1940.

Amano, H. and Daoust, R. *J. Histochem. Cytochem.*, **9**, 161, 1961.

Ambrose, E. J. Henry Ford International Symposium: *Biological Interactions in Normal and Neoplastic Growth* (Eds Brennan J. M. and Simposi W. L.), Churchill, London, 1962.

Anderson, P. J. and Song, S. K. *J. Neuropath. exp. Neurol.*, **21**, 274, 1962.

Andreussi, L. G. and Restelli-Fondelli, A. *Acta neurochir. (Wien)*, **15**, 40, 1966.

Ansell, G. B. and Richter, D. *Biochem. J.*, **57**, 70, 1954.

Ansell, G. B. and Dohmen, H. *J. Neurochem.*, **2**, 1, 1957.

Ansell, G. B. and Spanner, S. *J. Neurochem.*, **4**, 325, 1959.

Antoni, N. *Über Rückenmarkstumoren u. Neurofibrome*, Bergman Verlag, München, 1920.

Appel, S. H., Alpers, D. H. and Tomkins, G. M. *J. molec. Biol.*, **11**, 12, 1965.

Appel, S. H.: *Nature (Lond.)*, **213**, 1253, 1967.

Armstrong, M. D., McMillen, A. and Shaw, K. N. F. *BBA*, **25**, 422, 1957.

Arnaiz, G. R. de L. and de Robertis, E. D. P. *J. Neurochem.* **11**, 213, 1964.

Asp, N. G. *Biochem. J.*, 121, 299, 1971.

11

Augusti-Tocco, G. and Sato, G. *Proc. nat. Acad. Sci. (Wash.)*, **66**, 160, 1969.
Augustinsson, K. B. *Nature (Lond.)*, **181**, 1786, 1958.
Augustinsson, K. B. *Acta chem. scand.* **12**, 1150, 1959.
Augustinsson, K. B. *Ann. N. Y. Acad. Sci.*, **94**, 753, 1961.
Augustinsson, K. B. and Brody, S. *Clin. chim. Acta*, **7**, 560, 1962.
Awapara, J. and Seale, B. *J. biol. Chem.*, **194**, 497, 1952.
Awapara, J., Sandman, R. P. and Hanly, C. *Biochem. biophys. Acta (Amst.)*, **98**, 520, 1962.
Axelrod, J. *Science, N. Y.*, **126**, 400, 1957.
Axelrod, J. and Tomchick, R. *J. biol. Chem.*, **233**, 702, 1958.
Axelrod, J. and Laroche, J. M. *Science, N. Y.*, **130**, 800, 1959.
Axelrod, J. *J. biol. Chem.*, **237**, 1657, 1962.
Axelrod, J. *Science, N. Y.*, **140**, 499, 1963.
Axelrod, J. and Lerner, A. B. *BBA*, **71**, 650, 1963.
Axelrod, J. *Pharmacol. Rev.*, **18**, 95, 1966.
Axelrod, J. Mueller, R. A., Henry, J. P. and Stephens, P. M. *Nature (Lond.)*, **255**, 1059, 1970.
Azarnoff, D. I., Curran, G. L. and Williamson, W. P. *J. nat. Cancer Inst.*, **21**, 1109, 1958.
Bacq, Z. M., Gosselin, L., Dresse, A. and Renson, J. *Science, N. Y.*, **130**, 453, 1959.
Bailey, P. *Intracranial Tumours*, Charles C. Thomas, Springfield, Illinois, 1933.
Balázs, R. *Biochem. J.*, **86**, 494, 1963.
Balázs, R. and Cocks, W. A. *J. Neurochem.*, **14**, 1035, 1967.
Baltimore, D. *Nature (Lond.)*, **226**, 5252, 1970.
Banga, I., Ochoa, S. and Peters, R. A. *Biochem. J.*, **33**, 1980, 1939.
Barondes, S. H. and Cohen, H. D. *Science, N. Y.*, **151**, 594, 1966.
Barondes, S. H. and Cohen, H. D. *Proc. nat. Acad. Sci. (Wash.)* **58**, 157, 1967.
Barron, K. D., Bernsohn, J. and Hess, A. R. *J. Histochem. Cytochem.*, **9**, 656, 1961.
Barron, K. D., Bernsohn, J. and Hess, A. R. *J. Histochem. Cytochem.*, **11**, 139, 1963.
Barron, K. D., Bernsohn, J. and Hess, A. R. *J. Histochem. Cytochem.*, **12**, 42, 1964.
Bauer, H. J. *Symposium über den Liquor cerebrospinalis* (Ed. E. Seitelberger), Springer Verlag, Wienna, 1966, p. 166.
Bauer, H., Munz, E., Müller, D. and Meulen, V. *Second International Meeting of the International Society for Neurochemistry* (Eds R. Paoletti, R. Fumagalli, and C. Galli), Tamburini, Milan suppl., 1969.
Beaufay, H., Berleur, A. M. and Doyen, A. *Biochem. J.*, **66**, 32P, 1957.
Becker, N. H., Goldfischer, S., Shin, W. and Novikoff, A. B. *J. biophys. biochem. Cytol.* **8**, 649, 1960.
Beer, C. T. and Quastel J. H. *Can. J. Biochem. Physiol.*, **36**, 543, 1958.
Bell, J. L. and Baron, D. N. *Biochem. J.*, **82**, 5P, 1962.
Belpaire, F. and Laduron, P. *Biochem. Pharmac.*, **17**, 411, 1968.
Benda, P., Lightbody, J., Sato, G., Levine, L. and Sweet, W. *Science, N. Y.*, **161**, 370, 1968.
Benitez, H. X., Murray, M. and Woolley, D. W. *Anat. Rec.*, **121**, 446, 1955.
Bennetts, H. W., and Chapman, F. E. *Aust. vet. J.*, **13**, 138, 1937.
Benuck, M., Stern, F. and Lajtha, A. *J. Neurochem.* **17**, 1133, 1970.
Bergmann, F., Wilson, I. B. and Nachmansohn, D. *BBA*, **6**, 217, 1950.
Bergmann, F. and Rimon, S. *Biochem. J.*, **70**, 339, 1958.
Bergmann, F., Segal, R. and Rimon, S. *Biochem. J.*, **67**, 481, 1957.
Berl, S. and Waelsch, H. *J. Neurochem.*, **3**, 161, 1958.
Bernsohn, J., Barron, K. D. and Hess, A. R. *Proc. Soc. exp. Biol. Med.*, **108**, 71, 1961.
Bernsohn, J., Barron, K. D. and Hess, A. R. *Nature (Lond.)*, **195**, 285, 1962.
Bernsohn, J. and Barron, K. D. In *Variation in Chemical Composition of the Nervous System* (Ed. G. B. Ansell), Pergamon Press, Oxford, 1965, p. 12.
Bernsohn, J., Barron, K. D., Doolin, P. F., Hess, A. R. and Hedrick, M. T. *J. Histochem. Cytochem.*, **14**, 455, 1966.
Berry, J. F., Cavallos, W. H. and Wade, R. R. *J. Amer. Oil. Chem. Soc.*, **42**, 492, 1965.
Blake, A. and Peacocke, A. R. *J. Polym. Sci.*, **6**, 122, 1968.
Blaschko, H. *Pharmac. Rev.*, **18**, 39, 1966.

Blunt, M. J. and Wendell-Smith, C. P. *Nature*, *(Lond.)*, **216**, 605, 1967.
Bodansky, O. *Cancer*, *N. Y.*, **7**, 1191, 1200, 1954.
Bodansky, O. *Cancer*, *N. Y.*, **9**, 1087, 1956.
Bogoch, S., Rajam, P. C. and Belval, P. C. *Nature (Lond.)*, **204**, 73, 1964.
Bogoch, S. *Protides biol. Fluids*, **15**, 131, 1967.
Bogoch, S. *Second International Meeting of the International Society for Neurochemistry* (Eds R. Paoletti, R. Fumagalli and G. Galli), Tamburini, Milan, 1969, p. 97.
Bonavita, V. and Guarneri, R. *J. Neurochem.*, **10**, 755, 1963.
Bondy, S. C. and Roberts, S. *Biochem. J.*, **109**, 533, 1968.
Bondy, S. C., Roberts, S. and Morelos, B. S. *Biochem. J.*, **119**, 665, 1970.
Boxer, G. E. and Chonk, C. E. *Cancer Res.*, **20**, 85, 1960.
Boyd, J. W. *Biochem. J.*, **81**, 434, 1962.
Brachet, J. *C. R. Soc. Biol. (Paris)*, **133**, 88, 1940.
Bradham, L. S., Holt, A. D. and Sims, M. *BBA*, **201**, 250, 1970.
Brady, R. O. *J. biol. Chem.*, **235**, 3099, 1960.
Brante, G. *Acta physiol. scand.*, **18**. Suppl. 63, 1949.
Brodie, B. B., Kuntzman, R., Hirsch, C. W. and Costa, E. *Life Sci.*, **1**, 81, 1962.
Brody, T. M. and Bain, J. *J. biol. Chem.*, **195**, 685, 1952.
Brody, I. A., Resnik, J. S. and Engel, W. K.: *Arch. Neurol.*, **13**, 126, 1965.
Brookes, P. and Lawley, P. D. *Biochem. J.*, **80**, 496, 1961.
Brown, G. W., Chaikoff, Jr. I. L. and Chapman, D. D. *Proc. Soc. expt. Biol. Med.*, **84**, 586, 1953.
Brown, G. W., Jr., Katz, J. and Chaikoff, I. L. *Cancer. Res.*, **16**, 364, 1956.
Brownstein, M. J. and Heller, A. *Science, N. Y.*, **162**, 367, 1968.
Brox, L. W., Lacke, A. G., Gracy, R. W., Adelman, R. C. and Horecker, B. L. *Biochem. biophys. Res. Commun.*, **36**, 994, 1969.
Bruns, F. H., Jacob, W. and Weverinek, F. *Clinica Chim. Acta*, **1**, 63, 1956.
Brzin, M., Tennyson, V. M. and Duffy, P. E. *J. cell Biol.*, **31**, 315, 1966.
Bücher, Th. and Klingenberg, M. *Angew. Chem.*, **70**, 552, 1958.
Buckell, M. and Robertson, M. C. *Brit. J. Cancer*, **19**, 83, 1965.
Bülbring, E., Philpot, F. and Bosanquet, F. D. *Lancet*, **1**. 865, 1953.
Burgen, A. S. V. and Chipman, L. M. *J. Physiol.*, **114**, 296, 1951.
Burkard, W. P. and Gey, K. F. *Second International Meeting of the International Society for Neurochemistry* (Eds R. Paoletti, R. Fumagalli and G. Galli), Tamburini, Milan, 1969., p. 113.
Burstone, M. S. *J. natn. Cancer Inst.*, **16**, 1149, 1956.
Burton, R. M.: *The Neurochemistry of Nucleotides and Amino Acids.* (Ed. R. O. Brady), John Wiley, New York, 1960, p. 51.
Busch, H. and Nair, P. V.: *J. biol. Chem.*, **229**, 377, 1957.
Büttger, H. W., Scarlate, G., Müller, W. and Kemali, D. *Dtsch. Z. Nervenheilk.*, **176**, 67, 1957.
Cain, C. E., Bell, E. O., Jr., White, H. B., Jr., Sulya, L. L. and Smith, R. R. *BBA*, **144**, 493, 1967.
Calva, E., Loevenstein, J. M. and Cohen, P. P. *Cancer Res.*, **19**, 101, 605, 1959.
Canelas, H. M., De Jorge, F. B., Pereira, W. C. and Salum, J. *J. Neurochem.*, **15**, 1455, 1968.
Carneiro, J. and Leblond, C. P. *Science N. Y.*, **129**, 391, 1959.
Carruthers, C. *Cancer Res.*, **10**, 255, 1950.
Casamajor, L. *Arch. Histol. histopath. Arb. Großhirnrinde, Nissl. Arb.*, **6**, 52, 1918.
Cavanagh, J. B., Thompson, R. H. S. and Webster, G. K. *Quart. J. exp. Physiol.*, **39**, 185, 1954.
Chance, B. and Hess, B. *Science, N. Y.*, **129**, 700, 1959.
Chason, J. L., Landers, J. W., Gonzalez, J. E. and Brueckner, G. *J. Neuropath. exp. Neurol.*, **22**, 471, 1963.
Chirigos, M. A., Greengard, P. and Udenfriend, S. *J. biol. Chem.*, **235**, 2075, 1960.
Christensen Lou, H. O. and Clausen, J. *J. Neurochem.*, **15**, 263, 1968.
Christensen Lou, H. O., Clausen, J. and Biering, F. *J. Neurochem.*, **12**, 619, 1965.
Chytil, F.: *Biochem. biophys. Res. Commun.*, **19**, 630, 1965.
Clark, C. T., Weissbach, H. and Udenfriend, S. *J. biol. Chem.*, **210**, 139, 1954.

Clark, R. B. and Perkins, J. P. *Proc. nat. Acad. Sci. (Wash.)*, **68**, 2757, 1971.

Clausen, J. *Proceedings of the Thirteenth Colloquium of Bruges* (Ed. H. Peters), Elsevier, Amsterdam, 1966, p. 85.

Clitherow, J. W., Mitchard, M. and Harper, M. J. *Nature (Lond.)*, **199**, 1000, 1963.

Clouet, D. H. and Richter, D. *J. Neurochem.*, **3**, 219, 1959.

Cohen, L. H. *Fed. Proc.*, **16**, 165, 1957.

Cohen, M. D. *J. Neuropath. exp. Neurol.*, **14**, 70, 1955.

Cohen, S. R. *Handbook of Neurochemistry* (Ed. A. Lajtha), vol. 3, Plenum Press, New York, 1970, p. 87.

Collins, G. G. S. and Southgate, J. *Biochem. J.*, **117**, 38P, 1970.

Cori, G. T., Colowick, S. P. and Cori, C. F. *J. biol. Chem.*, **123**, 375, 1938.

Corridori, F., Cremona, T. and Tagliabue, G. *J. Neurochem.*, **6**, 142, 1960.

Couerbe, J. P. *Ann Chim. Phys.*, **56**, 160, 1834.

Crabtree, H. G. *Biochem. J.*, **23**, 536, 1929.

Craddock, V. M. *Nature (Lond.)*, **228**, 1264, 1970.

Crane, R. K. and Sols, A.: *J. biol. Chem.*, **123**, 375, 1953.

Criss, W. E. *Cancer Res.*, **31**, 1523, 1971.

Crout, J. R. *Pharmac. Rev.*, **18**, 651, 1966.

Cumings, J. N. *Brain*, **66**, 316, 1943.

Cumings, J. N. *Brain*, **73**, 244, 1950.

Cumings, J. N. *J. Neurol. Neurosurg. Psychiat.*, **16**, 152, 1953.

Cumings, J. N., Goodwin, H., Woodward, E. M. and Curzon, J. *J. Neurochem.*, **2**, 289, 1958.

Cumings, J. N. *Heavy Metals and the Brain*, Blackwell, Oxford, 1959.

Cumings, J. N. *IV. International Congress of Neuropathology* (Ed. H. Jacob), Vol. I, G. Thieme Verlag, Stuttgart, 1962, p. 157.

Cummins, J. and Hydén, H. *BBA*, **60**, 271, 1962.

Cutler, W. P., Watters, G. V. and Barlox, C. F. *Arch. Neurol.*, **11**, 225, 1964.

Dagnall, P. *Clinica Chim. Acta*, **2**, 381, 1957.

Das, P. K. and Liddel, J. *Biochem. J.*, **116**, 875, 1970.

Davies, W. E. *J. Neurochem.*, **17**, 397, 1970.

Davis, D. D. *Nature (Lond.)*, **231**, 153, 1971.

Davis, B. J. *Ann. N. Y. Acad. Sci.*, **121**, 404, 1964.

Davis, R. H., Copenhaver, J. H. and Carver, M. J. *J. Neurochem.*, **19**, 473, 1972.

Davison, A. N., Dobbing, J., Morgan, R. S. and Payling, Wright, G. *J. Neurochem.*, **3**, 89, 1958.

Davison, A. N., Dobbing, J., Morgan, R. S. and Payling Wright, G. *Lancet*, **1**, 658, 1959.

Davison, A. N. *Neurocytochemistry*, (Ed. C. W. M. Adams) Elsevier, Amsterdam, 1965, p. 189.

Dawson, D. M., Godfriend, T. L. and Kaplan, N. O. *Science, N. Y.*, **143**, 929, 1964.

Dawson, D. M. *J. Neurochem.*, **14**, 939, 1967.

Dawson, G., Kemp, S. F., Stoolmiller, A. C. and Dorfman, A. *Biochem. biophys. Res. Commun.*, **44**, 687, 1971.

Le Duve, C., Pressman, B. C., Gianetto, R., Wattiaux, R. and Appelmans, F. *Biochem. J.*, **60**, 604, 1955.

Le Duve, C. *Subcellular Particles* (Ed. Hayashi, T.), Ronald Press, N. Y., 1959, p. 128.

De Duve, C. *Lysosomes* (Ed. G. Wolstenholm), CIBA Foundation, London, 1963, p. 1.

De Lamirande, G., Daoust, R. and Cantero, A. *Can. Cancer, Conf.*, **4**, 43, 1961.

Delbrück, A., Zebe, E. and Bücher, T. *Biochem. Z.*, **331**, 273, 1959.

Dencker, S. J., Brönnestam, R. and Swahn, B. *Neurology*, **11**, 441, 1961.

De Risio, C. and Cumings, J. N.: *Riv. Neurobiol.*, **6**, 535, 1960.

De Robertis, E., Rodriguez, de Lores Arnaiz, G., Salganikoff, L., Pellegrino de Iraldi, A. and Zieher, L. M. *J. Neurochem.*, **10**, 225, 1963.

De Robertis, E., P. de Iraldi, de Lores Arnaiz, G. R. and Salganikoff, L. *J. Neurochem.*, **9**, 23, 1962.

De Robertis, E., Arnaiz, G. R. D. L., Alberici, A., Butcher, R. W. and Sutherland, E. W. *J. biol. Chem.*, **242**, 3487, 1967.

Derry, D. M. and Wolfe, L. S. *Science*, **158**, 1450, 1967.

Deul, D. H. and Van Breeman, J. F. L. *Clinica Chim. Acta*, **10**, 276, 1964.
De Vellis, J. and Inglish, D. *J. Neurochem.*, **15**, 1061, 1968.
De Vellis, J. and Inglish D.: *Second International Meeting of the International Society for Neurochemistry* (Eds R. Paoletti, R. Fumagalli and C. Galli), Tamburini, Milan, 1969, p. 151.
Dévényi, T., Rogers, S. J. and Wolfe, R. G. *Biochem. biophys. Res. Commun.*, **23**, 496, 1966.
Dewey, M. M. and Conklin, J. L. *Proc. Soc. exp. Biol. (N. Y.)*, **105**, 492, 1960.
Dickens, F. and Glock, G. E. *Biochem. J.*, **50**, 81, 1951.
Dingle, J. T. and Barrett, A. J. *J. Biochem.*, **109**, 19P, 1960.
Dingman, W. and Sporn, M. B. *J. Neurochem.*, **4**, 148, 1959.
di Prisco, G. *Pyridine Nucleotide-Dependent Dehydrogenase*. (Ed. H. Sund,) Springer Verlag, Berlin, 1970, p. 305.
Dixon, K. C. *Biol. Rev.*, **12**, 431, 1937.
Dohr, H. *Acta Neurochir.*, **9**, 543, 1961.
Dohr, H. and Herranz, M. P. *Klin. Wschr.*, **42**, 244, 1964.
Dohr, H., Menn, H., Herranz, P. and Mauteca, A. *Klin. Wschr.*, **44**, 407, 1966.
Dorfman, A. and Pei-Lee Ho *Proc. nat. Acad. Sci. (Wash.)*, **66**, 495, 1970.
Drabkin, D. L. *J. biol. Chem.*, **182**, 317, 1950.
Dravid, A. R. and Burdman, J. A. *J. Neurochem.*, **15**, 25, 1968.
Druckrey, H., Ivankovic, S. and Preussmann, R. *Z. Krebsforsch.*, **66**, 389, 1965.
Dubbs, C. A., Vivonia, C. and Heilburn, J. M. *Science, N. Y.*, **131**, 1529, 1960.
Du Bois, K. P. and Potter, V. R. *Cancer Res.*, **2**, 290, 1942.
Dulbecco, R. *Sci. Am.*, **216**, No. 4, 28, 1967.
Earle, K. M. *Lab. Invest.*, **8**, 66, 1959.
Ecobichon, D. J. and Kalow, W. *Biochem. Pharmacol.*, **11**, 573, 1962.
Ecobichon, D. J. *Can. J. Biochem.* **44**, 225, 1277, 1966.
Elliott, K. A. C. and Greig, M. E. *Biochem. J.*, **32**, 1407, 1938.
Engelhardt, V. A. and Sakov, N. E. *Biokhimiya*, **8**, 8, 1943.
Eppenberger, H. M., Eppenberger, M. E. and Scholl, A. *FEBS Symposium*, **18**, 269, 1970.
Eränkö, O., Kokko, A. and Söderholm, V. *Nature (Lond.)*, **193**, 778, 1962.
Ernster, L. *FEBS Symposium*, **17**, 1, 1969.
Essner, E. *J. biophys. biochem. Cytol.*, **7**, 329, 1960.
Falck, B. *Acta physiol. scand.*, **56**, Suppl. 197, 1962.
Falconer, I. R. *Mammalian Biochemistry*, Churchill, London, 1969.
Farron, F., Hsu, H. H. T. and Knox, W. E. *Cancer Res.* **32**, 302, 1972.
Feigen, J. and Wolf, A. *J. Neuropath. exp. Neurol.*, **17**, 522, 1958.
Feigen, I. and Wolf, A. *Arch. Path.*, **67**, 670, 1959.
Fellman, J. H. *Enzymologia*, **20**, 366, 1959.
Fewster, M. E. and Mead, J. F. *J. Neurochem.*, **15**, 1041, 1968.
Fidler, I. J. *Nature (Lond.)*, **229**, 564, 1971.
Fildes, R. A. and Parr, C. W. *Nature (Lond.)*, **201**, 89, 1963.
Fildes, R. A. and Harris, H. *Nature (Lond.)*, **209**, 261, 1966.
Filipowitz, W., Vincendon, G., Mandel, P. and Gombos, G. *Life Sci.*, **7**, 1243, 1968.
Fischer, W. and Müller, E. *Enzymol. Biol. & Clin.*, **11**, 450, 1970.
Fishman, W. H. *Enzymes* (Eds J. B. Sumner and K. Myrbäck), Vol. I, Academic Press, N. Y., 1950, p. 635.
Fishman, H. W. *Adv. Enzymol.*, **16**, 361, 1955.
Fishman, W. H. and Mitchell, G. W. *Ann. N. Y. Acad. Sci.*, **83**, 105, 1959.
Fishman, J. S. and Hayashi, M.: *J. Histochem. Cytochem.*, **10**, 515, 1962.
Fleisher, G. A., Wakim, K. G. and Goldstein, N. P. *Proc. Mayo Clin.*, **32**, 188, 1957.
Fleisher, G. A., Potter, C. S. and Wakim, K. G. *Proc. Soc. exp. Biol. N. Y.*, **103**, 229, 1960.
Folch, J. and Lees, M. *J. biol. Chem.*, **191**, 807, 1951.
Foldes, F. F., Zsigmond, E. K., Foldes, V. M. and Erdős, E. G. *J. Neurochem.*, **9**, 559, 1962.
Fonnum, F. *J. Biochem.*, **106**, 401, 1968.
Friede, R. L. *Virchows Arch. path. Anat. Physiol.*, **328**, 469, 1956.

Friede, R. L. *Virchows Arch. path. Anat. Physiol.*, **330**, 574, 1957.
Friede, R. L. *Virchows Arch. path. Anat. Physiol.*, **332**, 216, 1959.
Friede, R. L. *J. cell. Biol.*, **20**, 5, 1964.
Frieden, C. *J. biol. Chem.*, **234**, 815, 809, 2891, 1959.
Frieden, C. *J. biol. Chem.*, **238**, 3286, 1963.
Friedman, S. and Kaufman, S. *J. biol. Chem.*, **240**, 552, 1965.
Friend, C. and Wróblewski, F. *Science, N. Y.*, **124**, 173, 1956.
Fritz, I. B. and Yue, K. T. N. *Adv. Lipid Res.*, **4**, 279, 1963.
Frontali, N. *Acta chem. scand.*, **13**, 390, 1959.
Fruton, J. S. and Simmonds, S. *General Biochemistry*, John Wiley, New York, 1958.
Fujinaga, K., Parsons, J. Th., Beard, J. W., Beard, D. and Green, M. *Proc. nat. Acad. Sci. (Wash.)*, **67**, 1432, 1970.
Fukada, T. and Koelle, G. B. *J. biophys. biochem. Cytol.*, **5**, 433, 1959.
Fumagalli, R., Grossi, E., Paoletti, P. and Paoletti, R. *J. Neurochem.*, **11**, 561, 1964.
Fumagalli, R., Paoletti, R., Allegranza, A. and Paoletti, P. *Excerpta med. (Amst.)*, 1965.
Fumagalli, R., Grossi, E., Paoletti, P. and Paoletti, R. *J. Neurochem.*, **13**, 1005, 1966.
Furmanski, P., Silverman, D. J. and Lubin, M. *Nature (Lond.)*, **233**, 413, 1971.
Gaffney, P. J. *Biochem. J.*, **110**, 12P, 1968.
Gaitonde, M. K. and Richter, D. *Biochem. J.*, **59**, 690, 1955.
Gallo, R. C., Yang, S. S. and Ting, R. C. *Nature (Lond.)*, **228**, 927, 1970.
Gantt, R. R., Stromberg, K. J. and Montes de Oca, F.: *Nature (Lond.)*, **234**, 35, 1971.
Gatt, S. and Racker, E. *J. biol. Chem.* **234**, 1015, 1959.
Geiger, A., Magnes, J., Taylor, R. M. and Veralli, M. *Amer. J. Physiol.*, **177**, 138, 1954.
Geiger, R. S. *Fed. Proc.*, **16**, 44, 1957.
Gerhardt, W., Clausen, J., Christensen, E. and Riishede, J. *Acta neurol. scand.*, **39**, 85, 1963.
Gerhardt, W., Clausen, J. and Andersen, H. *Acta neurol. scand.*, **39**, 31, 1963a.
Giacobini, E. *J. Histochem. Cytochem.*, **8**, 419, 1960.
Giacobini, E. *J. Neurochem.*, **9**, 169, 1962.
Giarman, N. J., Friedman, D. and Picard-Ami, L. *Nature (Lond.)*, **186**, 480, 1960.
Giuditta, A. and Singer, T. P. *J. biol. Chem.*, **234**, 666, 1959.
Glassman, E. *A. Rev. Biochem.*, **38**, 605, 1969.
Glenner, G. C., Burtner, H. J. and Brown, G. W., Jr. *J. Histochem. Cytochem.*, **5**, 591, 1957.
Glenner, G. C., Burstone, M. S. and Meyer, D. B. *J. nat. Cancer Instr.*, **23**, 857, 1959.
Glock, G. E. and McLean, P. *Biochem. J.*, **56**, 171, 1954.
Glock, G. E. and McLean, P. *Biochem. J.*, **61**, 388, 1955.
Glock, G. E. and McLean, P. *Biochem. J.*, **65**, 412, 1957.
Gluszcz, A. *Acta Neuropathol.*, **3**, 184, 1963.
Gluszcz, A. and Giernat, L. *Folia Histochem. Cytochem.*, **7**, 15, 1969.
Gluszcz, A. and Giernat, L. *Folia Histochem. Cytochem.*, **8**, 191, 1970.
Gmelin, L. *Hoppe-Seylers Z. physiol. Chem.*, **1**, 118, 1826.
Godlewski, H. G. *Folia Histochem. Cytochem.*, **1**, Suppl. 1, 156, 1963.
Gold, P., Gold, M. and Freedman, S. O. *Cancer Res.*, **28**, 1331, 1968.
Goldberg, A. G., Takahura, K. and Rosenthal, K. L. *Nature (Lond.)*, **211**, 41, 1966.
Goldstein, F. B. *BBA*, **33**, 583, 1959.
Goldstein, M. *Pharmacol. Rev.*, **18**, 77, 1966.
Goldstein, M., Anagosta, B. and Goldstein, M. N. *Science, N. Y.*, **160**, 767, 1968.
Gomori, G. *Proc. Soc. exp. Biol. N. Y.*, **42**, 23, 1939.
Gomori, G. *Microscopic Histochemistry*, University Press, Chicago, 1952, p. 215.
Gomori, G. *Tex. Rep. Biol. Med.*, **13**, 636, 1955.
Gopal, K., Grossi, E., Paoletti, P. and Paoletti, R. *Acta neurochir.*, **11**, 333, 1963.
Gorkin, V. Z. *Pharmacol. Rev.*, **18**, 115, 1966.
Gottesfeld, J. M., Adams, N. H., El-Badry, A. M., Moses, V. and Calvin, M. *BBA*, **228**, 365, 1971.
Grahame-Smith, D. G. *BBA*, **86**, 176, 1964.
Grahame-Smith, D. G. *Biochem. biophys. Res. Commun.*, **16**, 586, 1964.
Grahame-Smith, D. G. *Biochem. J.*, **105**, 35,1 1967.

Graschenkov, N. I. and Hekht, B. M. *Exp. Neurol.*, **2**, 573, 1960.

Grasso, A., Cicero, T. and Moore, B. W. *Second International Meeting of the International Society for Neurochemistry* (Eds R. Paoletti, R. Fumagalli and C. Galli), Tamburini, Milan, 1969, p. 201.

Gray, G. M. *Biochem. J.*, **86**, 350, 1963.

Green, D. E. *Biochem. J.*, **30**, 2095, 1936.

Green, J. B., Oldewurtel, H. A., O'Doherty, D. S., Forster, F. M. and Sanchez-Longo, L. P. *Neurology (Minneap.)*, **7**, 313, 1957.

Green, J. B., Oldewurtel, H. A., O'Doherty, D. S. and Foster, F. M. *Arch. Neurol. Psychiat. (Chic.)*, **80**, 148, 1958.

Green, J. B., Oldewurtel, H. A. and Forster, F. M. *Neurology (Minneap.)*, **9**, 540, 1959.

Green, J. B. and Perry, M. *Neurology (Minneap.)*, **13**, 924, 1963.

Greengard, O., Smith, M. A. and Ács, G. *J. biol. Chem.*, **238**, 1548, 1963.

Greengard, P.: *Ann. N. Y. Acad. Sci.*, **185**, 18, 1971.

Greenstein, J. P. and Thompson, J. W. *J. nat. Cancer Inst.*, **4**, 271, 1943.

Greenstein, J. P., Eschenbrenner, A. P. and Leuthardt, F. M. *J. nat. Cancer Inst.* **5**, 55, 1944.

Greenstein, J. P. *Biochemistry of Cancer*, Academic Press, New York, 1954.

Griffin, A. C. *Advanc. Enzyme Regul.*, **3**, 361, 1964.

Grimm, F. C. and Doherty, M. D. *J. biol. Chem.*, **236**, 1980, 1961.

Grossi, E., Paoletti, P. and Paoletti, R. *Arch. int. Physiol. Biochem.*, **66**, 64, 1958.

Grossi, E., Paoletti, P. and Paoletti, R. *J. Neurochem.*, **6**, 73, 1960.

Grundig, E., Czitober, H. and Schobel, B. *Clin. Chim. Acta*, **12**, 157, 1965.

Gugler, R., Knuppen, R. and Breuer, H. *BBA*, **220**, 10, 1970.

Güttler, F. *Protides biol. Fluids*, **15**, 167, 1967.

Güttler, F. and Clausen, J. *Biochem. J.*, **114**, 839, 1969.

Haber, B., Kuriyama, K. and Roberts, E. *Biochem. Pharmac.*, **19**, 1119, 1970.

Haber, B., Kuriyama, K. and Roberts, E. *Science, N. Y.*, **168**, 598, 1970a.

Hagen, P. *Br. J. Pharmacol. chemother.*, **18**, 175, 1962.

Haije, W. G. and de Jong, M. *Clinica Chim. Acta*, **8**, 620, 1963.

Hajós, F. and Kerpel-Fronius, S. *Second International Meeting of the International Society for Neurochemistry.* (Eds R. Paoletti, R. Fumagalli and C. Galli), Tamburini, Milan, 1969, p. 265.

Hajra, A. K. and Radin, N. S. *J. Lipid Res.*, **4**, 448, 1963.

Haldar, D. *Biochem. biophys. Res. Commun.*, **40**, 129, 1970.

Harris, J. I., Meriwether, B. P. and Park, J. H. *Nature (Lond.)*, **197**, 154, 1963.

Harris, J. I. and Perham, R. N. *Nature (Lond.)*, **219**, 1025, 1968.

Hartmann, G., Behr, W., Beissner, K. A., Honikel, K. and Sippel, A. *Angew. Chem. Ausg. B.*, **7**, 693, 1968.

Hass, W. K. *Arch. Neurol. (Chic.)*, **14**, 443, 1966.

Hawthorne, J. N. *Biochem. J.*, **102**, 13P, 1966.

Heald, P. J. *Biochem. J.*, **67**, 529, 1957.

Hebb, C. O. and Whittaker, V. P. *J. Physiol.*, **142**, 187, 1958.

Heller, I. H. and Elliott, K. A. C. *Can. J. Biochem. Physiol.*, **32**, 584, 1954.

Heller, I. H. and Elliott, K. A. C. *Can. J. Biochem. Physiol.*, **33**, 395, 1955.

Hellung-Larsen, P. and Anderson, V. *FEBS Symposium*, **18**, 163, 1970.

Helmreich, E.: *FEBS Symposium*, **19**, 131, 1970.

Henderson, J. F. and Le Page, G. A. *Cancer Res.*, **19**, 887, 1959.

Hepp, D., Prusse, E., Weiss, H. and Wieland, P. *Advanc. Enzyme Regul.*, **4**, 89, 1965.

Hers, H. G. and Joassin, G. *Enzymol. Biol. & Clin.*, **1**, 4, 1961.

Herskovitz, J., Masters, C. J., Wasserman, P. M. and Kaplan, N. O. *Biochem. biophys. Res. Commun.*, **26**, 24, 1967.

Hess, R., Scarpelli, D. and Pearse, A. G. E. *J. biophys. biochem. Cytol.*, **4**, 753, 1958.

Hess, H. H. and Pope, A. *J. Neurochem.*, **5**, 207, 1960.

Hess, R. and Pearse, A. G. E. *BBA*, **71**, 285, 1963.

Hess, A. R., Angel, R. W., Barron, K. D. and Bernsohn, J. *Clin. chim. Acta*, **8**, 656, 1963a

Hess, H. H., Embree, L. J. and Shein, H. M. *Second International Meeting of the International Society for Neurochemistry* (Eds R. Paoletti, R. Fumagalli and C. Galli), Tamburini, Milan, 1969, p. 42.

Hilf, R., Goldenberg, H., Bell, C., Michel, I., Orlando, R. A. and Archer, F. L. *Enzymol. Biol. & Clin.*, **11**, 162, 1970.

Hill, B. R. and Levi, C. *Cancer Res.*, **14**, 513, 1954.

Hill, B. R. and Jordan, R. T. *Cancer Res.*, **17**, 144, 1957.

Himwich, H. E. *Brain Metabolism and Cerebral Disorders*, Williams and Wilkins, Baltimore, 1951, p. 185.

Hirs, C. H. W., Moore, S. and Stein, W. H. *J. biol. Chem.*, **235**, 633, 1960.

Hodgkin, W. E., Giblett, E. R., Levine, H., Bauer, W. and Motulsky, A. G. *J. clin. Invest.*, **44**, 486, 1965.

Hodson, A. W., Latner, A. L. and Raine, L. *Clin. chim. Acta*, **7**, 255, 1962.

Hofstal, B. H. J. *The Enzymes* (Eds P. D. Boyer, H. Lardy and K. Myrbäck), Academic Press, New York, 1960 vol. *4A*, 485.

Hogeboom, G. H. and Schneider, W. C. *Science, N. Y.*, **113**, 355, 1951.

Hokin, L. E. and Hokin, M. R. *BBA*, **18**, 102, 1955.

Hokin, L. E. and Hokin, M. R. *J. biol. Chem.*, **233**, 818, 822, 1958.

Hokin, L. E. and Hokin, M. R. *J. biol. Chem.*, **234**, 1387, 1959.

Holmberg, B. *Cancer Res.*, **21**, 1386, 1961.

Holmstedt, B. G. and Toschi, G. *Acta physiol. scand.*, **47**, 280, 1959.

Holstein, T. J. Fish, W. A. and Stokes, W. M. *J. Lipid Res.*, **7**, 634, 1966.

Holt, S. J. *Lysosomes* (Ed. G. Wolstenholm), Ciba Foundation, London, 1963, p. 114.

Holtz, P., Heise, R. and Lüdke, K. *Arch. exp. Path. Pharmak.*, **191**, 87, 1938.

Holtz, P. and Westermann, E. *Arch. exp. Path. Pharmak.*, **227**, 538, 1956.

Holzer, H., Mecke, D., Liess, K., Wulff, L., Heilmeyer, L., Ebner, E., Jr., Gancedo, C., Schutt, H., Battig, F. A., Heinrich, P. and Wolf, D. *FEBS Symposia*, **19**, 171, 1970.

Horecker, B. L. *J. biol. Chem.*, **183**, 593, 1950.

Horecker, B. L. and Smyrniotis, P. Z. *J. biol. Chem.*, **193**, 371, 1953.

Hsieh, K. M., Suntzeff, V. and Cowdry E. V. *Proc. Soc. exp. Biol. N. Y.*, **89**, 627, 1955.

Hsieh, K. M., Mac, S. S. and Sasananonth, K. *Cancer Res.*, **19**, 700, 1959.

Huszák, I. *Biochem. Z.*, **298**, 137, 1938.

Huszák, I. *Acta chem. scand.*, **1**, 813, 1947.

Hydén, H., Løvtrup, S. and Pigón, A. *J. Neurochem.*, **2**, 304, 1958.

Hydén, H. *Biochemistry of the Central Nervous System* (Ed. F. Brücke), Proc. of the Fourth International Congress of Biochemistry, Pergamon Press, Oxford, 1959, p. 64.

Hydén, H. and Pigón, A. *J. Neurochem.*, **6**, 57, 1960.

Hydén, H. *Neurochemistry* (Eds K. A. C. Elliott, I. H. Page and J. H. Quastel), Charles C. Thomas, Springfield, Illinois, 1962, p. 331.

Hydén, H. V. and Egyházi, E. *Proc. nat. Acad. Sci. (Wash.)*, **48**, 1366, 1962., 49, 618, 1963., 52, 1030, 1964.

Hydén, H. and Lange, P. W. *Proc. nat. Acad. Sci. (Wash.)*, **53**, 946, 1965.

Hydén, H. and Lange, P. W. *Science, N. Y.*, **159**, 1370, 1968.

Hydén, H. and Lange, P. W. *Proc. nat. Acad. Sci. (Wash.)*, **65**, 898, 1970.

Ibba, F. M. and Viale, G. L. *Oncologia*, **18**, 44, 1964.

Ikuta, F. and Zimmermann, H. M. *Archs Path.*, **78**, 377, 1964.

Inscoe, J. K., Daly, J. and Axelrod, J. *Biochem. Pharmac.*, **14**, 1257, 1965.

Itoh, C., Yoshinaga, K., Sato, T., Ishida, N. and Wada, Y. *Nature (Lond.)*, **193**, 477, 1962.

Jacob, F. and Monod, J. *J. molec. Biol.*, **3**, 318, 1961.

Jacob, F. and Monod, J. *Biochem. biophys. Res. Commun.*, **18**, 693, 1965.

Jacob, M., Stevenin, J., Jund, R., Judes, C. and Mandel, P. *J. Neurochem.*, **13**, 619, 1966.

Jacobs, H., Heldt, H. W. and Klingenberg, M. *Biochem. biophys. Res. Commun.*, **16**, 516, 1964.

Jacobs, H. K., Keutel, H. J., Yue, R. H., Okabe, K. and Kuby, S. A. *Fed. Proc.*, **27**, 640, 1968.

Jacobson, B. and Kaplan, N. O. *J. biol. Chem.*, **226**, 603, 1957.
Jacobson, K. B. and Kaplan, N. O. *J. biophys. biochem. Cytol.*, **1**, 31, 1957a.
Jamieson, D. *Biochem. Pharmacol.*, **12**, 693, 1963.
Jansz, H. S., Brons, D. and Warrings, M. G. P. J. *BBA*, **34**, 573, 1959.
Järnefelt, J. *BBA*, **48**, 104, 1961.
Johnson, A. C., McNabb, A. R. and Rossiter, R. J. *Biochemistry, N. Y.*, **44**, 494 1949.
Johnson, M. K. *Biochem. J.*, **82**, 281, 1962.
Joo, F. and Várkonyi, T. *Acta biol. Acad. Sci. hung.*, **20**, 359, 1969.
Jouvet, M. *Science, N. Y.*, **163**, 32, 1969.
Joyce, D. *Experimentia (Basel)*, **19**, 187, 1963.
Juul, P. *Clin. chim. Acta*, **19**, 205, 1968.
Kalckar, H. *J. biol. Chem.*, **148**, 127, 1943.
Kalow, W. and Staron, N. *Can. J. Biochem. Physiol.*, **35**, 1035, 1957.
Kalow, W. and Davies, R. O. *Biochem. Pharmacol.*, **1**, 185, 193, 1959.
Kamaryt, J. and Zazvorka, Z. *Clin. chim. Acta*, **9**, 559, 1964.
Kaplan, N. O., Colowick, S. P. and Neufeld, E. F. *J. biol. Chem.*, **205**, 1, 1953.
Kaplan, N. O. *Bact. Rev.*, **27**, 155, 1963.
Karcher, D., van Sande, M. and Lowenthal, A. *J. Neurochem.*, **4**, 135, 1959.
Kartha, G., Bellow, J. and Harker, D. *Nature (Lond.)*, **213**, 862, 1967.
Kasabjan, S. S. *Arkh. Patol.*, **13**, (2), 34, 1951.
Kates, J. R., Winterton, R. and Schlesinger, K. *Nature (Lond).*, **229**, 345, 1971.
Katona, F., Cholnoky, E., Szabó, Gy., Sáfár, M., Slowik, F. and Wollemann, M. Unpublished results 1965.
Kaufman, S., Gilvarg, C., Cori, O. and Ochoa, S. *J. biol. Chem.*, **203**, 869, 1953.
Kellner, B. *Z. Krebsforsch.*, **49**, 633, 1939.
Kennedy, E. P. and Weiss, S. B. *J. Amer. Chem. Soc.*, **77**, 250, 1955.
Kennedy, E. P. and Weiss, S. B. *J. biol. Chem.*, **222**, 193, 1956.
Kerr, S. E., Kfoury, G. A. and Hoddad, F. S. *BBA*, **84**, 461, 1964.
Kim, H. and D'Orio, A. *Can. J. Biochem.*, **46**, 295, 1968.
King, E. J. *Biochem. J.*, **25**, 799, 1931.
Kirsch, W. M. *Neurol. (Minneap.)*, **13**, 23, 1963.
Kirsch, W. *Second International Meeting of the International Society for Neurochemistry. Round Table Discussion on Neurochemistry of Brain Tumours* (Ed. P. Paoletti), Unione tipografica, Milan, 1969, p. 8.
Kit, S. *Amino Acids, Proteins, and Cancer Biochemistry* (Ed. J. T. Edsall), Academic Press, New York, 1960, p. 147.
Kitto, G. B., Stolzenbach, F. E. and Kaplan, N. O. *Biochem. biophys. Res. Commun.*, **38**, 31, 1970.
Klavins, J. V., Mesa-Tejada R. and Weiss, N. *Nature, New Biology.*, **234**, 153, 1971.
Klein, J. R., Hurwitz, R. and Olsen, N. S. *J. biol. Chem.*, **164**, 509, 1946.
Klein, J. R., Hurwitz, R. and Olsen, N. S. *J. biol. Chem.*, **167**, 1, 1947.
Klein, D. C., Berg, G. R., Weller, J. and Glinsmann, W. *Science, N. Y.*, **167**, 1738, 1970.
Klenk, E. *Z. Phys. Chem.*, **302**, 268, 1955.
Klingenberg, M. and Slencza, W. *Biochem. Z.*, **331**, 334, 1959.
Koe, B. K. and Weissman A., *J. Pharmacol. exp. Ther.*, **154**, 499, 1966.
Koelle, G. B. *J. comp. Neurol.*, **100**, 211, 1954.
Koelle, G. B. *J. Pharmacol. exp. Ther.*, **114**, 167, 1955.
Koelle, G. B. *J. Pharmacol. exp. Ther.*, **103**, 153, 1951.
Koenig, H. *J. biophys. biochem. Cytol.*, **4**, 785, 1958.
Koenig, H. and Barron, K. D. *J. Neuropath. exp. Neurol.*, **22**, 336, 1963.
Koenig, H., Gaines, D., McDonald, T., Gray, R. and Scott, J. *J. Neurochem.*, **11**, 729, 1964.
Komma, D. J. *J. Histochem. Cytochem.*, **11**, 619, 1963.
Kornberg, A. and Pricher, W. E. *J. biol. Chem.*, **189**, 125, 1951.
Kornberg, A. and Horecker, B. L. *Methods in Enzymology* (Eds S. P. Colowick and N. O. Kaplan), Vol. II, Academic Press, New York, 1953, p. 323.
Kornberg, A. and Pricher, W. E. *J. biol. Chem.*, **204**, 329, 345, 1953a.
Kostič, D. and Buchheit, F. *Life Sci.*, **9**, 589, 1970.

Koszalka, T. R., Horne, S., Schlegel, B. and Altman, K. I. *BBA*, **35**, 197, 1959.
Kraml, J., Koldovský, O., Heringová, A., Jirsová, V. and Kácl, K. *FEBS Symposium*, **18**, 263, 1970.
Krebs, H. A. *Biochem. J.*, **29**, 1951, 1935.
Krebs, H. A. and Eggleston, L. V. *Biochem. J.*, **34**, 442, 1940.
Krebs, H. A. *Biochem. J.*, **47**, 605, 1950.
Krebs, H. A. and Hems, R. *BBA*, **12**, 172, 1953.
Krebs, H. A. and Veech, R. L. *FEBS Symposium*, **17**, 101, 1969.
Kreuzberg, G. W., Minauf, M. and Gullotta, F. *Histochemie*, **6**, 8, 1966.
Kreuzberg, G. W. and Gullotta, F. *Z. ges. Neurol. Psychiat.*, **209**, 378, 1967.
Krupka, R. M. *Biochemistry, N. Y.*, **5**, 1988, 1966.
Krupka, R. M. *Biochemistry, N. Y.*, **6**, 1183, 1967.
Kubowitz, F. and Ott, P. *Biochemistry, N. Y.*, **314**, 94, 1943.
Kunitz, M. J. *J. gen. Physiol.*, **24**, 15, 1940.
Kunitz, M. *Science*, **108**, 19, 1948.
La Brosse, E. H., Axelrod, J., Kopin, I. J. and Kety, S. S. *J. clin. Invest.*, **40**, 253, 1961.
Laduron, P. and Belpaire, F. *Biochem. Pharmac.*, **17**, 1127, 1968.
Lagnado, J. R. and Hardy, M. *Variation in Chemical Composition of the Nervous System* (Ed. G. B. Ansell), Pergamon Press, Oxford, 1965, p. 63.
Laird, A. K. and Barton, A. D. *Science, N. Y.*, **124**, 32, 1956.
Lajtha, A., Furst, S., Gerstein, A. and Waelsch, H. *J. Neurochem.*, **1**, 289, 1957.
Lajtha, A. *J. Neurochem.*, **2**, 209, 1958.
Lajtha, A. *Regional Neurochemistry* (Eds S. S. Kety and J. Elkes), Pergamon Press, Oxford, 1961, p. 26.
Lajtha, A. and Marks, N. *Diseases Nerv. Syst. GWAN* Suppl., **30**, 36, 1969.
La Motta, R. V., Babbott, D. and Wetstine, H. *J. Cancer. Res.*, **21**, 249, 1961.
La Motta, R. V., McComb, R. B., Noll, C. R. Jr., Wetstone, H. J. and Reinfrank, R. F. *Arch. Biochem. Biophys.*, **124**, 299, 1968.
La Motta, R. V., Woronick, C. L. and Reinfrank, R. F. *Arch. Biochem. Biophys.*, **136**, 448, 1970.
Landow, H., Kabat, E. A. and Newman, W. *Arch. Neurol. Psychiat.* (*Chic.*), **48**, 518, 1942.
Lange, C. F. and Kohn, P. *Cancer Res.*, **21**, 1055, 1961.
Langvad, F. *Int. J. Cancer*, **3**, 17, 1968.
Lantos, P. L. *Experientia* (*Basel*), **27**, 1322, 1971.
Lapham, L. W. *J. Neuropath. exp. Neurol.*, **18**, 244, 1959.
Larner, J. *J. biol. Chem.*, **202**, 491, 1953.
Larrabee, M. G., Klingman, J. D. and Leicht, W. S. *J. Neurochem.*, **10**, 549, 1963.
Lawley, P. D. *Progr. Nucl. Acid Res. & molec. Biol.*, **5**, 89, 1966.
Lazarus, S. S., Wallace, B. J., Edgar, G. W. F. and Volk, B. W. *J. Neurochem.*, **9**, 227, 1962.
Lehmann, H. and Ryan, E. *Lancet*, **11**, 124, 1956.
Lehmann, H. and Silk, E. *Nature (Lond.)*, **193**, 561, 1964.
Lehrer, G. M. in *The Biology and Treatment of Intracranial Tumors* (Eds W. S. Fields and P. C. Sharkey), Charles C. Thomas, Springfield, Illinois, 1962, p. 14.
Lehrer, G. M. *IV. International Congress of Neuropathology*. Proceedings Vol. I. (Ed. H. Jacob), G. Thieme Verlag, Stuttgart, 1962a, p. 66.
Lenta, M. P. and Riehl, M. A. *Cancer Res.*, **12**, 498, 1952.
Le Page, G. A. *Cancer Res.*, **8**, 193, 1948.
Lerman, L. S. *Proc. nat. Acad. Sci. (Wash.)*, **49**, 94, 1963.
Leshovaia, N. N. *Biokhimiya*, **19**, 478, 1954.
Leuzinger, W. and Baker, A. L. *Proc. nat. Acad. Sci. (Wash.)*, **57**, 446, 1967.
Leuzinger, W., Goldberg, M. and Cauvin, E. *J. molec. Biol.*, **40**, 217, 1969.
Levan, G., Mitelman, F., Nichols, W. W., Beckman, G. and Beckman, L. *Hereditas* (*Lund*), **68**, 143, 1971.
Levi-Montalcini, R. *Harvey Lectures*, Academic Press, New York, 1965, p. 217.
Levin, E. Y. and Kaufman, S. *J. biol. Chem.*, **236**, 2043, 1961.
Levvy, G. A. *Biochem. J.*, **52**, 464, 1952.
Lipcina, L. P. *Vop. Neurockir.*, **16**, (3), 30, 1952.

Loewenstein, W. R. *Sci. Amer.*, **222**, (5), 78, 1970.

Logan, J. E., Mannell, W. A. and Rossiter, R. J. *Biochem. J.*, **51**, 470, 1952.

Lovenberg, W., Jequier, E. and Sjoerdsma, A. *Science, N. Y.*, **155**, 217, 1967.

Lowenthal, A., van Sande, M. and Karcher, D. *Ann. N. Y. Acad. Sci.*, **94**, 988, 1961.

Lowenthal, A., Karcher, D. and van Sande, M. *J. Neurochem.*, **11**, 247, 1964.

Lowenthal, A. *Symposium über den Liquor cerebrospinalis* (Ed. Feitelberger), Springer Verlag, Wienna, 1966. p. 121.

Lowry, O. H. *Physiol. Rev.*, **32**, 431, 1952.

Lowry, O. H., Roberts, N. R., Wu, M. L., Hixon, W. S. and Crawford, E. J. *J. biol. Chem.*, **207**, 19, 1954.

Lowry, O. H., Roberts, N. R. and Lewis, C. *J. biol. Chem.*, **220**, 879, 1956.

Lowry, H. O. and Passoneau, J. V. *Biochem. Pharmacol.*, **9**, 173, 1962.

Lucas-Lenard, J. and Lipmann, F. *Science, N. Y.*, **57**, 1050, 1967.

Lundin, L. G. and Allison, A. C. *BBA*, **127**, 527, 1966.

Luse, S. A. *Biology and Treatment of Intracranial Tumors*, Charles C. Thomas, Springfield, Illinois, 1962, p. 79.

Lynen, F. *Proc. Int. Symposium on Enzyme Chemistry*, Tokyo and Kyoto, 1958, p. 259.

MacNair, Scott, D. B., Pakoskey, A. M. and Sanford, K. K. *J. natn. Cancer Inst.*, **25**, 1365, 1960.

MacNair, Scott, D. B., Morris, A. L., Reiskin, A. B. and Pakoskey, A. M. *Cancer Res.*, **22**, 857, 1962.

Mahaley, S. *Second International Meeting of the International Society for Neurochemistry. Round Table Discussion on Neurochemistry of Brain Tumours.* (Ed. P. Paoletti) Unione tipografica, Milan, 1969.

Mahler, H. R., Raw, I., Molinary, R. and Ferreira do Amaral, D. *J. biol. Chem.*, **233**, 230, 1958.

Mahler, H. R., Moore, W. J. and Thompson, R. J. *J. biol. Chem.*, **241**, 1283, 1966.

Maio, J. J. and Rickenberg, H. V. *BBA*, **37**, 101, 1960.

Maker, H. S., Lehrer, G. M., Silides D. J. and Weiss, C.: *Ann. N. Y. Acad. Sci.*, **159**, 461, 1969.

Mandell, A. J. and Morgan, M. *Nature (Lond.)*, **227**, 75, 1970.

Mandell, A. J. *Biochemistry of Brain and Behaviour*, Plenum Press, New York, 1970, p. 97.

Mango, C., Suguira, K. and Wróblewski, F. *Cancer Res.*, **18**, 682, 1958.

Mann, K. G. and Vestling, C. S. *Biochemistry, N. Y.*, **9**, 3020, 1968.

Manno, N. J., McGuckin, W. F. and Goldstein, N. P.: *Neurology (Minneap.)*, **15**, 49, 1965.

Mansour, T. E. *Pharmacol. Rev.*, **18**, 173, 1966.

Mardashev, S. R. and Mamaeva, V. V. *Biokhimiya*, **15**, 478, 1950.

Marinesco, G. *Ann. Anat. path.*, **5**, 233, 1928.

Markert, C. L. and Moller, F. *Proc. nat. Acad. Sci. (Wash.)*, **45**, 753, 1959.

Marks, N. and Lajtha, A. *Biochem. J.*, **89**, 438, 1963.

Marks, N. and Wollemann, M. Unpublished results, 1964.

Martin, A. J. P. and Porter, R. R. *Biochem. J.*, **49**, 215, 1951.

Masurovsky, E. B. and Noback, C. R. *Nature (Lond.)*, **200**, 847, 1963.

Matakas, F. *Dtsch. Z. Nervenheilk.*, **196**, 287, 1969.

Matsushima, T., Kawabe, S., Shibuya, M. and Sugimira, T. *Biochem. biophys. res. Commun.*, **30**, 565, 1968.

Mayor, S. J. *Science, N. Y.*, **166**, 1165, 1969.

McConnel, J. V., Jacobson, A. L. and Kimble, D. P. *J. comp. Physiol. Psychol.*, **52**, 1, 1959.

McDonald, R., Gibson G. and Thorn, M. B. *Biochem. J.*, **114**, 775, 1969.

McEwen, B. S. and Hydén, H. *Proceedings of the NATO Advanced Study Institute*, (Ed. O. Wallas) Vol. I, Academic Press, New York, 1965, p. 131.

McEwen, B. S. and Hydén, H. *J. Neurochem.*, **13**, 823, 1966.

McEwen, B. S. and Hydén, H. *Molecular Basis of Some Aspects of Mental Activity* (Ed. O. Wallas). Vol. I, Academic Press, New York, 1967, p. 131.

McIlwain, H. *Biochemistry of the Central Nervous System.* J. A. Churchill, London, 1959, p. 65.

Mellorn, A. and Tappel, A. L. *J. Lipid Res.*, **8**, 479, 1967.
Mendel, B. and Rudney, H. *Biochem. J.*, **37**, 59, 1943.
Menten, M. L., Junge, J. and Green, M. H. *J. biol. Chem.*, **153**, 471, 1944.
Merril, C. R., Geier, M. R. and Petricciani, J. C. *Nature (Lond.)*, **233**, 398, 1971.
Meyerhof, O. and Geliazkova, N. *Arch. Biochem.*, **12**, 405, 1947.
Meyerhof, O. and Wilson, J. R. *Arch. Biochem.*, **17**, 153, 1948.
Meyer-Ruge, W. *Z. Krebsforsch.*, **68**, 276, 1966.
Michaelson, A. *Ann. N. Y. Acad. Sci.*, **144**, 387, 1967.
Miller, F. P., Maickel, R. P. and Cox, R. H. Jr. *Biochem. Pharmacol.*, **19**, 435, 1970.
Molinoff, P. B., Brimijoin, S., Weinshilboum, R. and Axelrod, J. *Proc. nat. Acad. Sci. (Wash.)*, **66**, 453, 1970.
Monier, R., Zajdela, F., Chaix, P. and Petit, J. F. *Cancer. Res.*, **19**, 927, 1959.
Monis, B., Banks, B. M. and Rutenburg, A. M. *Cancer*, **13**, 386, 1960.
Monod, J., Wyman, J. and Changeux, J. P. *J. molec. Biol.*, **12**, 88, 1965.
Monseau, G. and Cumings, J. N. *Neurol. Neurosurg. Psychiat.*, **28**, 56, 1965.
Moore, B. W. *Biochem. biophys. Res. Commun.*, **19**, 739, 1965.
Moran, J. F., Sourkes, T. L. and Chavez, B. *Can. J. Biochem. Physiol.*, **41**, 2376, 1963.
Moran, J. F. and Sourkes, T. L. *J. Pharmacol. (Fr.)*, **148**, 252, 1965.
Morrison, L. R. and Zamecnik, P. C. *Archs Neurol. Psychiatr. (Chic.)*, **63**, 367, 1950.
Morton, R. K. *Biochem. J.*, **60**, 573, 1955.
Moss, D. W. and King, E. J. *Biochem. J.*, **84**, 192, 1962.
Mossakowski, M. J. *J. Neuropath. exp. Neurol.*, **21**, 137, 1962.
Mueller, R. A., Thoenen, H. and Axelrod, J. *Molec. Pharmacol.*, **5**, 463, 1969.
Mueller, R. A., Thoenen, H. and Axelrod, J. *Science, N. Y.*, **158**, 468, 1969a.
Müller, W. and Nasu, H. *Frankf. Z. Path.*, **70**, 417, 1960.
Müller, W. and Nasu, H. *Naturwissenschaften*, **49**, 496, 1962.
Myers, D. K., Tol, J. W. and De Junge, M. H. T. *Biochem. J.*, **65**, 223, 1957.
Nachlas, M. M. and Seligman, A. M. In Gomori, G. *Microscopic Histochemistry*, Univ. of Chicago Press, Chicago, 1952, p. 203.
Nagatsu, T., Levitt, M. and Udenfriend, S. *J. Biol. Chem.*, **239**, 2910, 1964.
Nagy, A., Róna, E., Katona, F. and Wollemann, M. *Enzyme*, **12**, 467, 1971.
Naidoo, D. and Pratt, O. E. *J. Neurol. Neurosurg. Psychiatry*, **14**, 287, 1951.
Nasu, H. and Viale, G. L. *IV. International Congress of Neuropathology. Proceedings*, Vol. I. G. Thieme Verlag, Stuttgart, 1962, p. 115.
Nasu, H. *Dtsch. Z. Nervenheilk.*, **185**, 67, 1964.
Nayyar, N. *Neurology (Minneap.)*, **13**, 287, 1963.
Nelson, P., Ruffner, W. and Nirenberg, M. *Proc. nat. Acad. Sci. (Wash.)*, **66**, 160, 1969.
Nicholas, H. J. and Thomas, B. E. *BBA*, **36**, 583, 1959.
Nicholas, H. J. and Bombaugh, K. J. *BBA*, **98**, 372, 1965.
Nievel, J. G. and Cumings, J. N. *Nature (Lond.)*, **214**, 1123, 1967.
Nigam, V. N., MacDonald, H. L. and Cantero, A. *Cancer Res.*, **22**, 131, 1962.
Nirenberg, M. W. *J. biol. Chem.*, **234**, 3088, 1959.
Norton, and Podulso, *J. Lipid Res.*, **12**, 84, 1971.
Novikoff, A. B. *Cell Physiology of Neoplasm.* (Ed. T. Hsu) G. Univ. Texas Press, 1960, p. 219.
O'Brien, R. L., Olenick, J. G. and Hahn, F. E. *Proc. nat. Acad. Sci. (Wash.)*, **55**, 1511, 1966.
Ochoa, S. *J. biol. Chem.*, **174**, 115, 1948.
Ochoa, S. *Advanc. Enzymol.*, **15**, 183, 1954.
O'Connor, J. S. and Laws, E. R. *Arch. Neurol.*, **9**, 91, 1963.
Oesterle, W., Kamig, K., Büchel, W. and Nickel, A. K. *J. Neurochem.*, **17**, 1403, 1970.
Ogawa, K. and Zimmermann, H. M. *J. Histochem. Cytochem.*, **7**, 342, 1959.
Ono, T., Blair, D. G. R., Potter, V. R. and Morris, H. P. *Cancer Res.*, **23**, 240, 1963.
Ord, M. G. and Thompson, R. N. S. *Biochem. J.*, **51**, 245, 1952.
Osske, G., Werzok, R. and Jänisch, W. *Naturwissenschaften*, **55**, 495, 1968.
Osterberg, K. A. and Wattenberg, L. W. *Arch. Neurol.*, **7**, 211, 1962.
Ostrowski, W., Wasyl, Z., Weber, M., Guminka, M. and Luchter, E. *BBA*, **221**, 297, 1970.

Otani, T. T. and Morris, H. P. *Advanc. Enzyme Regul.*, **3**, 325, 1965.
Owen, O. E., Morgan, A. P., Kemp, H. G., Sullivan, J. M., Herrera, M. G. and Cahill, G. F. *J. clin. Invest.*, **46**, 1589, 1967.
Palladin, A. V. and Poljakova, M. N. *Dokl. Akad. Nauk SSSR*, **107**, 568, 1956.
Paoletti, P., Visca, A. and Villani, R. *Minerva med. (Roma)*, **52**, 590, 1961.
Paoletti, P. *Ric. scient.*, **3**, 413, 1963.
Paoletti, R., Fumagalli, R., Grossi, E. and Paoletti, P. *J. Amer. Oil chem. Soc.*, **42**, 400, 1965.
Parmar, S. S., Sutter, M. C. and Nickerson, M. *Can. J. Physiol. & Pharmacol.*, **39**, 1335, 1961.
Pasternak, G. A. *Biochemistry of Differentiation*, John Wiley, London, 1970.
Pasteur, L. *Études sur la bière*, Gautiers-Villars, Paris, 1876.
Paxton, H. D. *Neurol. (Minneap.)*, **9**, 376, 1959.
Pearse, A. G. E. *Histochemistry. Theoretical and Applied*, Churchill, London, 1961.
Penhoet, E., Rajkumar, T. and Rutter, W. J. *Proc. nat. Acad. Sci. (Wash.)*, **56**, 1275, 1966.
Pepler, W. J. and Pearse, A. G. E. *J. Neurochem.*, **1**, 193, 1957.
Perria, L., Viale, G., Ibba, F., Andreussi, L. and Viale, E. *Neuropsichiatria*, **20**, 3, 1964.
Pietruczko, R. and Theorell, H. *Arch. Biochem. Biophys.*, **131**, 288, 1969.
Pinter, I. *Acta physiol. Acad. Sci. hung.*, **11**, 39, 1957.
Pitillo, R. F. and Hunt, D. E. *Antibiotics. I. Mechanism of Action* (Eds D. Gottlieb and P. D. A. Shaw). Springer Verlag, New York, 1967, p. 481.
Pletscher, A., Besendorf, H., Bächtold, H. P. and Gey, K. F.: *Helv. physiol. pharmacol. Acta*, **17**, 202, 1959.
Polgár, L. *Acta physiol. Acad. Sci. hung.*, **25**, 308, 1964.
Pollack, M. A., Taylor, J. and Williams, R. *J. Cancer Res.*, **2**, 739, 1942.
Pope, A., Hess, H. H. and Allen, N. *Prog. Neurobiol.*, **2**, 216, 1957.
Porter, H. and Folch, J. *Arch. Neurol. Psychiat.*, **77**, 8, 1957.
Potanos, J. N., Wolf, A. and Cowen, D. *J. Neuropath. exp. Neurol.*, **18**, 627, 1959.
Potter, V. R. and Busch, H. *Cancer Res.*, **10**, 353, 1950.
Potter, L. and Axelrod, J. *Pharmac. exp. Ther.*, **142**, 299, 1963.
Prasad, K. N. and Hsie, A. W. *Nature, New Biology*, **233**, 141, 1971.
Promyslov, M. S.: *Nature (Lond.)*, **210**, 1279, 1966.
Promyslov, M. S.: *Second International Meeting of the International Society for Neurochemistry. Round Table Discussion on Neurochemistry of Brain Tumours* (Ed. R. Paoletti), Unione tipografica, Milan, 1969, p. 4.
Prostenik, A. and Munk-Weinert, M. *BBA*, **71**, 732, 1963.
Pullmann, A. and Pullmann, B. *Cancérisation par les substances chimiques et structures moléculaire*, Masson et Cie, Paris, 1965.
Quastel, J. H. *Physiol. Rev.*, **19**, 135, 1939.
Quastel, J. H. and Zatman, L. J. *BBA*, **10**, 256, 1953.
Racker, E. *Advanc. Enzymol.*, **15**, 141, 1954.
Racker, E. *Advanc. Enzymol.*, **15**, 173, 1959.
Racker, E., Wu, R., Alpers, Y. B. and Edsall, J. T. *Amino Acids, Proteins and Cancer Biochemistry*, Academic Press, New York, 1960, p. 175.
Ragland, J. B. *Biochem. biophys. Res. Commun.*, **31**, 203, 1968.
Räihä, N. C. R. and Koskinen, M. S. *Life Sci.*, **3**, 1091, 1964.
Raskin, N. H. and Sokoloff, L. *Science, (N.Y.)* **162**, 131, 1968.
Raspail, F. V. *Ann. Sci. Nat.*, **6**, 384, 1825.
Reich, E. and Goldberg, I. H. *Prog. Nucleic Acid Res. Mol. Biol.*, **3**, 183, 1964.
Reinafarje, B. and Potter, V. R. *Cancer Res.*, **13**, 49, 1957.
Reiner, L., Rutenberg, A. M. and Seligman, A. M. *Cancer, N. Y.*, **10**, 563, 1957.
Ressler, N., Olivero, E., Thompson, G. R. and Joseph, R. R. *Nature (Lond.)*, **210**, 695, 1966.
Rhian, M. and Potter, V. R. *Cancer Res.*, **7**, 714, 1947.
Richter, D., Gaitonde, M. K. and Cohn, P. *Structure and Function of the Cerebral Cortex* (Eds D. B. Tower and J. P. Schadé), Elsevier, Amsterdam, 1960, p. 340.
Roberts, E. and Tschikoff, G. H. *Science, N. Y.*, **109**, 14, 1949.

Roberts, E., Tanaka, K. K., Tanaka, T. and Simondsen, D. G. *Cancer Res.*, **16**, 970, 1956.
Roberts, R. B., Flexner, J. B. and Flexner, L. B. *Proc. nat. Acad. Sci. (Wash.)*, **66**, 310, 1970.
Robertson, W. and Kahler, H. J. *J. nat. Cancer Inst.*, **2**, 595, 1942.
Robins, E., Smith, D. E. and Jen, M. K. *Ultrastructure and Cellular Chemistry of Neural Tissue* (Ed. Paul B. Hoebner), New York, 1957, p. 205.
Robinson, J. C. and Pierce, J. E. *Nature (Lond.)*, **204**, 472, 1964.
Robinson, G. A., Butcher, R. W. and Sutherland, E. W. *A. Rev. Biochem.*, **37**, 149, 1968.
Rodriguez De Lores Arnaiz G. and De Robertis, E. *J. Neurochem.*, **11**, 213, 1964.
Róna, E., Nagy, A. and Wollemann, M.: *Biochemistry and Histochemistry of Cerebral Tumours*. International Symposium of the Associations of Polish Neuropathologists and Polish Neurological Society, Commission of Neurochemistry (Ed. M. Wender), Poznan, 1971, p. 45.
Róna, E., Nagy, A., Wollemann, M. and Slowik, F. *Neuropath. Pol.* **10**, 207, 1972.
Rose, S. P. R.: *Second International Meeting of the International Society for Neurochemistry* (Eds R. Paoletti, R. Fumagalli, C. Galli), Tamburini, Milan, 1969, p. 45.
Rosenberg, R. N., Vandeventer, L., De Francesco, L. and Friedkin, M. E. *Proc. nat. Acad. Sci. (Wash.)*, **58**, 1436, 1971.
Rosenthal, O., Bowie, M. A. and Wagoner, G. *Science, N. Y.*, **92**, 382, 1940.
Rubinstein, L. J., Klatzo, I. and Miquel, J. *J. Neuropath. exp. Neurol.*, **21**, 116, 1962a.
Rubinstein, L. J. and Smith, B. *Nature (Lond.)*, **193**, 895, 1962.
Rubinstein, L. J. and Sutton, C. H. *J. Neuropath. exp. Neurol.*, **23**, 196, 1964.
Rubinstein, L. J., Scheinberg, L. C. and Levy, W. A. *J. Neuropath. exp. Neurol.*, **24**, 155, 1966.
Russel, D. S., Rubinstein, L. J. and Lumsden, C. E. *Pathology of Tumours of the Nervous System*, Edward Arnold, London, 1963, p. 281.
Rutter, W. J., Richards, O. C., Woodfin, H. M. and Weber, C. S. *Advanc. Enzyme Regul.*, **1**, 39, 1963.
Sacks, W. *J. appl. Physiol.*, **10**, 37, 1957.
Sacktor, B., Packer, L. and Estabrook, R. W. *Arch. Biochem. Biophys.*, **80**, 68, 1959.
Salganikoff, L. and De Robertis, E. *J. Neurochem.*, **12**, 287, 1965.
Samorajski, T. and McCloud, J. *Lab. Invest.*, **10**, 492, 1961.
Sanadi, D. R., Gibson, D. M., Ayengar, P. and Jacob, M. *J. biol. Chem.*, **218**, 505, 1956.
Sano, K., Chigasaki, H. and Takakura, K. *Proc. of the Third International Congress of Neurological Surgery, International Congress Series No. 110*. Excerpta Medica Found, Amsterdam, 1966, p. 575.
Saraswathi, S. and Bachhawat, B. K. *J. Neurochem.*, **13**, 237, 1966.
Sayde, F. W. and Hill, B. R. *Proc. Soc. exp. Biol., N. Y.*, **96**, 695, 1957.
Schade, A. L. *BBA*, **12**, 163, 1953.
Schiffer, D. and Vesco, C. *IV. International Congress of Neuropathology, Proceedings*, Vol. **I** (Ed. H. Jacob), G. Thieme Verlag, Stuttgart, 1962, p. 83.
Schlom, J., Spiegelman, S. and Moore, D. *Nature (Lond.)*, **231**, 97, 1971.
Schmidt, G. and Tannhauser, S. J. *J. biol. Chem.*, **161**, 83, 1945.
Schmitz, H., Hurlpert, R. B. and Potter, V. R. *J. biol. Chem.*, **209**, 41, 1954.
Schneider, W. C. and Potter, V. R. *J. biol. Chem.*, **149**, 217, 1943.
Schneider, W. C. and Hogeboom, G. H. *J. nat. Cancer Inst.*, **10**, 969, 1950.
Schneider, W. C. and Hogeboom, G. H. *Cancer Res.*, **11**, 1, 1951.
Schubert, D., Humphreys, S., Baroni, C. and Cohn, M. *Proc. nat. Acad. Sci. U.S.A.*, **66**, 160, 1970.
Schuberth, P. and Kreuzberg, G. *Histochemie*, **9**, 367, 1967.
Schwerin, P. Bessman, S. P. and Waelsch, H. *J. biol. Chem.*, **184**, 37, 1950.
Seeds, N. W., Gilman, A. G., Amano, T. and Nirenberg, M. W. *Proc. nat. Acad. Sci. (Wash.)*, **66**, 160, 1970.
Seifert, H. *Klin. Wschr.*, **44**, 469, 1966.
Sellinger, O. Z., Beaufay, H., Jacques, P., Doyen, A. and De Duve, C. *Biochem. J.*, **74**, 450, 1960.

Sellinger, O. Z. and de Verster, B. *J. biol. Chem.*, **237**, 2836, 1962.
Selverstone, B. and Moulton, M. *J. Brain*, **80**, 362, 1957.
Sen, A. K. and Tobin, T. *J. biol. Chem.*, **244**, 6596, 1969.
Shack, J. *J. biol. Chem.*, **226**, 573, 1957.
Shapira, F., Dreyfus, J. C. and Allard, D. *Clin. chim. Acta*, **20**, 439, 1968.
Shapira, F., Dreyfus, J. C. and Schapira, G. *Nature (Lond.)*, **200**, 995, 1963.
Shapiro, D. M., Dietrich, L. S. and Shils, M. E. *Cancer Res.*, **16**, 575, 1956.
Shaw, C. R., Syner, F. N. and Tashian, R. E. *Science, N. Y.*, **138**, 31, 1962.
Shaw, C. R. and Koen, A. L. *Science, N. Y.*, **140**, 70, 1963.
Shein, H. M. *Science, N. Y.*, **159**, 1476, 1968.
Shepherd, J. A. and Kalnitsky, G. *J. biol. Chem.*, **207**, 605, 1954.
Shervin, A. L., Leblanc, F. E. and McCann, W. P. *Arch. Neurol.*, **18**, 311, 1968.
Shimizu, H., Greveling, C. R. and Daly, J. *Proc. nat. Acad. Sci. (Wash.)*, **6**, 1033, 1970.
Shimizu, H., Tanaka, S., Suzuki, T. and Matsukado, Y. *J. Neurochem.*, **18**, 1157, 1971.
Shrivastava, G. C. and Quastel, J. H. *Nature (Lond.)*, **196**, 876, 1962.
Sibley, J. A. and Lehninger, A. D. *J. nat. Cancer Inst.*, **9**, 303, 1949.
Sibley, J. A., Fleischer, G. A. and Higgins, G. M. *Cancer Res.*, **15**, 306, 1955.
Sibley, J. A. *Ann. N. Y. Acad. Sci.*, **75**, 339, 1958.
Sjoerdsma, A. *Pharmacol. Rev.*, **11**, 374, 1959.
Sjoerdsma, A. *Pharmacol. Rev.*, **18**, 645, 1966.
Skou, J. C. *BBA*, **23**, 294, 1957.
Slagel, D. E., Dittmer, J. S. and Wilson, C. B. *J. Neurochem.*, **14**, 789, 1967.
Slagel, D. E., Wilson, C. B. and Simmons, P. G. *Ann. N. Y. Acad. Sci.*, **159**, 490, 1969.
Slater, T. F. *Biochim. biophys. Acta (Amst.)*, **77**, 365, 1963.
Smith, B. *Brain*, **86**, 89, 1963.
Smith, A. L., Satterwhite, S. H. and Sokoloff, L. *Science, N. Y.*, **163**, 79, 1969.
Smithies, O. *Biochem. J.*, **71**, 585, 1959.
Sottocasa, G. L., Kuylenstierna, B., Ernster, L. and Bergstrand, A. *J. cell. Biol.*, **32**, 415, 1967.
Sourkes, T. L. *Rev. Can. Biol.*, **17**, 328, 1958.
Sourkes, T. L. *Brit. Med. Bull.*, **21**, 66, 1965.
Sourkes, T. L. *Pharmacol. Rev.*, **18**, 53, 1966.
Spackman, D. H., Stein, W. H. and Moore, S. *J. biol. Chem.*, **235**, 1555, 1960.
Speck, J. F. *J. biol. Chem.*, **179**, 1405, 1949.
Spencer, N., Hopkinson, D. A., Harris, H. *Nature (Lond.)*, **204**, 742, 1964.
Spiegel-Adolf, M. and Wycis, H. T. *I. J. Neuropath. exp. Neurol.*, **12**, 601, 1954.
Spiegel-Adolf, M. and Wycis, H. T. *II. J. Neuropath. exp. Neurol.*, **16**, 404, 1957.
Spolter, P. D., Adelman, R. C. and Weinhouse, S. *J. biol. Chem.*, **240**, 1327, 1965.
Sporn, M. B. *Biochem. Pharmacol.*, **20**, 1029, 1971.
Squires, R. F. *Biochem. Pharmacol.*, **17**, 1401, 1968.
Stahl, W. L., Smith, J. C., Napolitano, L. M. and Basford, R. E. *J. cell. Biol.*, **19**, 293, 1963.
Standjord, P. E., Thomas, K. E. and White, L. P. *J. clin. invest.* **38**, 211, 1960.
Stedman, E. and Stedman, E. *Biochem. J.*, **29**, 2563, 1935.
Stein, A. A. and Eisinger, G. *J. Neuropath. exp. Neurol.*, **22**, 170, 1963.
Stein, A. A., Opalka, E. and Peck, F. *Arch. Neurol.*, **8**, 50, 1963.
Stewart, J. A. *Biochem. biophys. Res. Commun.*, **46**, 1405, 1972.
Stjärne, L. *Acta physiol. scand. Suppl.*, **62**, 228, 1964.
Stjärne, L., v. Euler and Lishajko, F. *Biochem. Pharmacol.*, **13**, 809, 1964.
Straub, M. *BBA*, **184**, 649, 1969.
Strecker, H. J. *Arch. Biochem. Biophys.*, **46**, 128, 1953.
Strickland, K. P. *Can. J. med. Sci.*, **30**, 484, 1952.
Strickland, K. P., Thompson, W., Subrahmanyam, D. and Rossiter, R. J. *Biochem. J.*, **87**, 128, 1963.
Studnitz, W. *Klin. Wschr.*, **40**, 163, 1962.
Sugimura, T., Sato, S., Kawabe, S., Suzuki, N., Chien, T. C. and Takakura, K. *Nature (Lond.)*, **222**, 1070, 1969.

Sugimura, T., Sato, S. and Kawabe, S. *Biochem. biophys. Res. Commun.*, **39**, 626, 1970.

Sur, K., Moss, D. W. and King, E. J. *J. Proc. Ass. clin. Biochem.*, **2**, 11, 1962.

Sutherland, V. C., Burbridge, T. N. and Elliott, H. W. *Amer. J. Physiol.*, **180**, 195, 1955.

Sutherland, E. W. and Rall, T. W. *J. biol. Chem.*, **237**, 1220, 1962.

Sutton, C. H. and Becker, N. H. *Ann. N. Y. Acad. Sci.*, **159**, 497, 1969.

Svenneby, G. *J. Neurochem.*, **17**, 1591, 1970.

Svennilson, E., Dencker, S. J. and Swahn, B. *Neurology*, **11**, 989, 1961.

Svensmark, O. and Kristensen, P. *BBA*, **67**, 441, 1963.

Svensmark, O. *Acta physiol. scand.*, **59**, 378, 1963.

Swahn, B., Brönnestam, R. and Dencker, S. J. *Neurology*, **11**, 437, 1961.

Szliwovski, H. B. and Cumings, J. N. *Brain*, **84**, 204, 1961.

Szybalski, W. and Iyer, V. N. *Antibiotics. I. Mechanism of Action* (Eds D. Gottlieb and P. D. Shaw), Springer Verlag, Berlin 1967, p. 211.

Tajima, T. *Acta Med. biol. (Niigata)*, **8**, 137, 1960.

Takeuchi, T. and Ohama, H. *Gann*, **49**, 240, 1958.

Tallan, H. H., Moore, S. and Stein, W. H. *J. biol. Chem.*, **211**, 915, 927, 1954.

Tallan, H. H., Moore, S. and Stein, W. H. *J. biol. Chem.*, **230**, 707, 1958.

Tani, E., Ametani, T., Higashi, N. and Fujihara, E. *Ultrastructure Res.*, **36**, 211, 1971.

Tanaka, R. and Abbod, G. L. *J. Neurochem.*, **10**, 7, 1962.

Tanford, C. and Hauenstein, J. D. *BBA*, **19**, 535, 1956.

Tashian, R. E. *Proc. Soc. exp. Biol. Med., N. Y.*, **108**, 364, 1961.

Tator, C. H. and Schwartz, M. L. *Second International Meeting of the International Society for Neurochemistry. Round Table Discussion on Neurochemistry of Brain Tumours.* (Ed. P. Paoletti), Unione tipografica, Milan, 1969.

Temin, H. M. and Mizutani, S. *Nature (Lond.)*, **226**, 1211, 1970.

Thoenen, H. *Nature (Lond.)*, **228**, 861, 1970.

Thompson, H. G., Hirschberg, E., Jr., Osnos, M. and Gelhorh, A. *Neurology*, **9**, 545, 1959.

Thorne, C. J. R., Grossmann, L. I. and Kaplan, N. O. *BBA*, **73**, 193, 1963.

Thorne, C. J. R. and Dent, N. J. *FEBS Symposium*, **18**, 203, 1970.

Thudichum, J. L. W. *A Treatise on the Chemical Constitution of the Brain*, Bailliere, Tindall and Cox, London, 1884.

Timmis, G. M. and Williams, D. F. *Chemotherapy of Cancer, the Antimetabolite Approach*, Butterworths, London, 1967.

Tomkins, G. M. and Yielding, K. L. *Cold Spring Harbor Symposia*, **24**, 331, 1961.

Tomkins, G. M., Gelehrter, Th. D., Granner, D., Martin, D., Samuels, H. H. Jr. and Thompson, E. B. *Science, N. Y.*, **166**, 1474, 1969.

Torack, R. M. and Barnett, R. J. *Neurol.*, **6**, 224, 1962.

Torack, R. M. and Barnett, R. J. *J. Neuropath. exp. Neurol.*, **23**, 46, 1964.

Tower, D. B. and Elliott, K. A. C. *J. appl. Physiol.*, **5**, 375, 1953.

Tower, D. B. *The Neurochemistry of Nucleotides and Amino Acids* (Eds R. O. Bray and D. B. Tower), John Wiley, New York, 1960, p. 173.

Tower, D. B. *Neurochemistry of Epilepsy*, Charles C. Thomas, Springfield, Illinois, 1960a.

Towne, J. C. *Nature (Lond.)*, **201**, 709, 1964.

Tsanev, R. *BBA*, **103**, 374, 1960.

Tsao, M. U. *Arch. Biochem. Biophys.*, **90**, 234, 1960.

Tuttle, J. P. and Wilson, J. E. *BBA*, **212**, 185, 1970.

Udenfriend, S., Zaltzman-Nirenberg, P. and Nagatsu, T. *Biochem. Pharmacol.*, **14**, 837, 1965.

Udvarhelyi, G. B., O'Connor, J. S., Walker, A. E., Laws, E. R. Jr. and Kranin, S. *IVth International Congress of Neuropathologic Proceedings*, Vol. I (Ed. H. Jacob) G. Thieme Verlag, Stuttgart, 1962, p. 95.

Ursing, B., Dencker, S. J. and Swahn, B. *Acta med. scand.*, **171**, 715, 1962.

Utley, J. D. *J. Neurochem.*, **10**, 423, 1963.

Vandenheuvel, F. A., Fumagalli, R., Paoletti, R. and Paoletti, P. *Life Sci.*, **6**, 439, 1967.

van der Helm, H. J. *Nature (Lond.)*, **194**, 773, 1962.

van Hoof, F. *FEBS Symposium*, **19**, 339, 1970.

van Kempen, G. M. J., Van der Berg, C. J., Van der Helm, H. J. and Veldstra, H. *J. Neurochem.*, **12**, 581, 1965.

Vauquelin, L. N. *Ann. chim.*, **31**, 37, 1811.

Vazquez, D., Staehelin, T., Celma, M. L., Battaner, E., Fernandez-Munoz, R. and Munro, R. E. *FEBS Symposium*, , **21**, 109, 1970.

Velick, S. F. and Hayes, J. E. *J. biol. Chem.*, **203**, 545, 1953.

Vessel, R. S. and Bearn, A. G. *Proc. Soc. exp. Biol. N. Y.*, **94**, 96, 1957.

Viale, G. L. and Ibba, F *Acta neurochir. (Wien)*, **12**, 475, 1964.

Viale, G. L. and Andreussi, L. G. *Acta neuropath.*, **4**, 538, 1965.

Viale, G. L., Kroh, H., Grosse, G. and Viale, E. *Second International Meeting of the International Society for Neurochemistry. Round Table Discussion on Neurochemistry of Brain Tumours* (Ed. P. Paoletti), Unione tipografica, Milan, 1969, p. 6.

Viale, G. L. and Kroh, H. *International Symposium on Biochemistry and Histochemistry of Cerebral Tumours* (Ed. M. Wender), Association of Polish Neuropathologists, Poznan, 1971, p. 64.

Victor, J. V. and Wolf, A. *Proc. Ass. Rev. nerv. ment. Dis.*, **16**, 44, 1937.

Vignais, P. V. and Vignais, P. M.: *BBA*, **47**, 515, 1961.

Villar-Palasi, C., Goldberg, N. D., Bishop, J. S., Nuttall, F. Q. and Larner, J. *FEBS Symposium*, **19**, 149, 1970.

Viveros, O. H., Arqueros, L., Connett, R. J. and Kirschner, N. *Molec. Pharmacol.*, **5**, 60, 1969.

Volk, M. E., Millington, R. H. and Weinhouse, S. *J. biol. Chem.*, **195**, 493, 1952.

Volkers, S. A. S. and Taylor, M. W. *Biochemistry*, **10**, 488, 1971.

Vorbrodt, A. *J. Histochem. Cytochem.*, **9**, 647, 1961.

Vos, J. and Van der Helm, H. J. *J. Neurochem.*, **11**, 209, 1967.

Voute, P. A. *Neuroblastoom, Ganglioneuroom, Phaechromocytoom*, A. Oosthoek's Uitgeversmaatschapij NV, Utrecht, 1968.

Waelsch, H. *Advanc. Enzymol.*, **13**, 237, 1952.

Waelsch, H. *Proc. of the Fourth International Congress of Biochemistry*, **3**, 36, 1959, Pergamon Press, New York.

Waksman, A. and Faenza, C. *Clin. Chim. Acta*, **5**, 450, 1960.

Waltimo, O. and Talanti, S. *Nature (Lond.)*, **205**, 499, 1965.

Warburg, O., Posener, K. and Negelein, E. *Biochem. Z.*, **152**, 309, 1924.

Warburg, O. *The Metabolism of Tumours*, Constable, London, 1930.

Warburg, O. and Christian, W. *Biochem. Z.*, **238**, 131, 1931.

Warburg, O. and Christian, W. *Biochemistry, N. Y.*, **314**, 299, 1942.

Warburg, O. and Hiepler, E. *Z. Naturf.*, **7b**, 193, 1952.

Warburg, O. *Science, N. Y.*, **124**, 296, 1956.

Ward, D. C., Reich, E. and Goldberg, I. H. *Science, N. Y.*, **149**, 1259, 1965.

Warecka, K. and Bauer, H. *J. Neurochem.*, **14**, 783, 1967.

Waring, M. J. *Symp. Soc. gen. Microbiol.*, **16**, 234, 1966.

Wattenberg, L. W. *Amer. J. Path.*, **35**, 113, 1959.

Webb, T. E. and Potter, R. V. *Cancer Res.*, **26**, 1022, 1966.

Webb, T. E. and Morris, H. P. *Biochem. J.*, **115**, 575, 1969.

Weber, G. and Cantero, A. *Cancer Res.*, **15**, 105, 1955.

Weber, G. and Cantero, A. *Cancer Res.*, **17**, 995, 1957.

Weber, G. and Morris, H. P. *Cancer Res.*, **23**, 987, 1963.

Weber, G. and Lea, M. A. *Advanc. Enzymol.*, **4**, 115, 1965.

Weber, G. *Naturwissenschaften*, **9**, 418, 1968.

Webster, G. R., Marples, E. A. and Thompson, R. H. S. *Biochem. J.*, **65**, 374, 1957.

Weinhouse, S. *Cancer Res.*, **31**, 1166, 1971.

Weissbach, H., Redfield, S. and Udenfriend, S. *J. biol. Chem.*, **229**, 953, 1957.

Weiss, B., Shein, H. M. and Snyder, R. *Life Sci.*, **10**, 1253, 1971.

Wender, M. and Walingóra, Ž. *IV. Internationaler Kongress für Neuropathologie* (Ed. H. Jacob), Vol. I. G. Thieme Verlag, Stuttgart, 1962.

Wender, M., Zgorzalewicz, B. and Huber, Z. *International Symposium on Biochemistry and Histochemistry of Cerebral Tumours*, Poznan (Ed. M. Wender), Association of Polish Neuropathologists, Poznan, 1971, p. 67.

Wenner, C. E., Spirtis, M. A. and Weinhouse, S. *Proc. Soc. exp. Biol. Med.*, **89**, 416, 1951.
Wenner, E., Spirtis, M. A. and Weinhouse, S. *Cancer Res.*, **12**, 44, 1952.
Wenner, C. E., Dunn, D. F. and Weinhouse, S. *Cancer Res.*, **12**, 44, 1952.
Wenner, C. E. and Weinhouse, S. *Cancer Res.*, **13**, 21, 1953.
West, E. S. and Todd, W. T. *Textbook of Biochemistry*, Macmillan, New York, 1956.
White, H. B. Jr. and Smith, R. R. *J. Neurochem.*, **15**, 293, 1968.
Whittaker, V. P. *Biochem. J.*, **72**, 694, 1959.
Wieland, T. and Pfleiderer, G. *Biochem. Z.*, **329**, 112, 1957.
Wieland, T. and Pfleiderer, G. *Angew. Chem.*, **1**, 169, 1962.
Wilson, I. P. and Ginsburg, S. *BBA*, **18**, 168, 1955.
Winkelmann, R. K.: *Cancer*, **13**, 626, 1960.
Wolf, A., Kabat, E. A. and Newman, W. *Amer. J. Path.*, **19**, 423, 1943.
Wolfe, L. S. and Lowden, J. A. *Can. J. Biochem.*, **42**, 1041, 1964
Wolfgram, F. and Rose, A. S. *Neurology*, **10**, 365, 1960.
Wollemann, M. and Feuer, G. *Acta physiol. Acad. Sci. hung.*, **10**, 446, 1956.
Wollemann, M. *Acta physiol. Acad. Sci. hung.*, **16**, 153, 1959.
Wollemann, M. and Zoltán, L. *Arch. Neurol.*, **6**, 161, 1962.
Wollemann, M. and Áfra, D. *Confinia neurol.*, **25**, 125, 1963.
Wollemann, M. and Dévényi, T. *Neurochem.*, **10**, 83, 1963.
Wollemann, M., Rubinstein, L. J., Sutton, G. I., Smith, J. C. and Foldes, F. F. *Variation in Chemical Composition of the Nervous System as Determined by Developmental and Genetic Factors*, (Ed. G. B. Ansell), Pergamon Press, Oxford, 1965.
Wollemann, M. *Recent Development of Neurobiology in Hungary*, Vol. I (Ed. K. Lissák), Akadémiai Kiadó, Budapest, 1967, p. 46.
Wollemann, M., Nagy, A., Katona, F. and Paraicz, E. *Second International Congress of the International Society for Neurochemistry* (Eds R. Paoletti, R. Fumagalli and C. Galli), Tamburini, Milan, 1969, p. 420.
Wollemann, M. *Métabolisme des Médiateurs Chimiques du Système Nerveux*, Masson et Cie, Paris; Akadémiai Kiadó, Budapest, 1970.
Wollemann, M. and Gazsó, L. *Symposium of the European Tissue Culture Society*, Budapest, 1971.
Wollemann, M., Gazsó, L. and Róna, E. *Neuropat. Pol.* **10**, 168, 1972.
Wollemann, M., Róna, E. and Katona, F.: *International Congress of Neurochemistry*, Budapest, 1971.
Wróblewski, F. and LaDue, J. S. *Proc. Soc. exp. Biol. Med.*, *N. Y.*, **90**, 210, 1955.
Wróblewsky, F. and Decker, B. *Amer. J. Clin. Path.*, **28**, 269, 1957.
Wróblewski, F. *Ann. N. Y. Acad. Sci.*, **75**, 322, 1958.
Wróblewski, F. and Gregory, K. F. *Ann. N. Y. Acad. Sci.*, **94**, 912, 1961.
Wu, R.: *Cancer Res.*, **19**, 1217, 1959.
Wu, R. and Racker, E. *J. biol. Chem.*, **234**, 1036, 1959.
Yanagihara, T. and Cumings, J. N. *Arch. Neurol.*, **19**, 241, 1968.
Yakulis, V. J., Gibson, C. W. and Heller, P. *Amer. J. clin. Path.*, **38**, 378, 1962.
Yamada, H., Yasunobo, K. T., Yamano, T. and Mason, H. S. *Nature (Lond.)*, **198**, 1092, 1963.
Yip, A. T. and Larner, J. *Phys. Chem. Physics.*, **1**, 383, 1969.
Yip, M. C. M. and Knox, W. E. *J. Biol. Chem.*, **245**, 2199, 1970.
Yonetani, T. *Biochem. biophys. Res. Commun.*, **3**, 549, 1960.
Youdim, M. B. H., Collins, C. G. S. and Sandler, M. *FEBS Symposium*, **18**, 281, 1970.
Youngstrom, K. A., Woodhall, B. R. and Graves, R. W. *Proc. Soc. exp. Biol. Med*, *N. Y.*, **48**, 555, 1941.
Yushok, W. D. *Cancer Research.*, **19**, 104, 1959.
Zacks, S. I. *Amer. J. Pathol.*, **34**, 293, 1958.
Zech, R. *Hoppe-Seylers Z. physiol. Chem.*, **350**, 1415, 1969.
Zeller, E. A. *Ann. N. Y. Acad. Sci.*, **80**, 551, 1959.
Zimmermann, H. and Arnold, H. *Cancer Res.*, **1**, 919, 1941.
Zlotnik, A. E., Weisenberg, E. and Chovers, I. *J. Lab. clin. Med.*, **54**, 207, 1959.
Zomzely, C. E., Roberts, S., Gruber, C. P. and Brown, D. M. *J. biol. Chem.*, **243**, 5396, 1968,
Zülch, K. J. *The Biology and Treatment of Intracranial Tumors*, (Eds W. S. Fields and P. C. Sharkey). Charles C. Thomas, Springfield, Illinois, 1962, p. 151.

INDEX